DYSPHAGIA COOKBOOK FOR NEWLY DIAGNOSED

Easy, Delicious and Nourishing Soft Foods Recipes

Peggy C. Valentine

Table of Contents

Chapter 1:

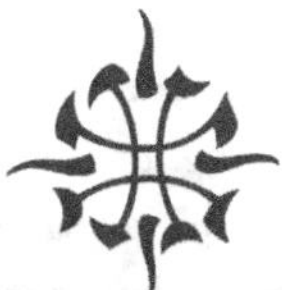

INTRODUCTION

An Overview of Dysphagia

Dysphagia is a medical condition that affects the ability to swallow. It can occur in individuals of all ages, from infants to the elderly, and can be caused by various factors. In this section, we will explore the fundamentals of dysphagia, its causes, symptoms, and potential complications.

At its core, dysphagia refers to difficulties or abnormalities in the swallowing process. Swallowing is a complex action involving the coordination of muscles and nerves in the mouth, throat, and esophagus. When this process is disrupted, individuals may experience discomfort, pain, or even the inability to swallow properly.

There are two main types of dysphagia: oropharyngeal and esophageal. Oropharyngeal dysphagia occurs when there are difficulties in the oral and pharyngeal stages of swallowing, which involve chewing, forming a bolus (a cohesive mass of food), and propelling it into the throat. Esophageal dysphagia, on the other hand, occurs when there are issues with the esophagus, the muscular tube that transports food from the throat to the stomach.

Dysphagia can arise from several causes. Neurological conditions, such as stroke, Parkinson's disease, or multiple sclerosis, can affect the nerves and muscles involved in swallowing. Structural abnormalities, such as strictures or tumors in the throat or esophagus, can also contribute to dysphagia.

Additionally, certain medical treatments, such as radiation therapy or surgeries in the head and neck area, may lead to swallowing difficulties.

Identifying dysphagia can be challenging, as its symptoms can vary. Common signs include coughing or choking during meals, feeling as though food is getting stuck in the throat, regurgitation, weight loss, and recurrent respiratory infections. If left untreated, dysphagia can lead to malnutrition, dehydration, aspiration pneumonia (when food or liquid enters the lungs), and a decreased quality of life.

Fortunately, there are various diagnostic methods and treatment options available for individuals with dysphagia. Medical professionals, such as speech-language pathologists and gastroenterologists, can conduct assessments to evaluate swallowing function. These assessments may include videofluoroscopy, in which X-ray imaging is used to observe the swallowing process, or fiberoptic endoscopic evaluation of swallowing (FEES), where a flexible scope is passed through the nose to examine the throat and larynx during swallowing.

Treatment for dysphagia depends on its underlying cause and severity. It can range from making dietary modifications, such as altering food textures or thickness, to exercises that strengthen swallowing muscles. In some cases, medications or surgical interventions may be necessary. Speech-language pathologists often play a crucial role in dysphagia management, providing swallowing therapy and strategies to improve safety and efficiency during mealtimes.

Tips for Managing Dysphagia in Daily Life

Living with dysphagia can present unique challenges, but with proper management strategies, individuals can navigate their daily lives more comfortably and reduce the risk of complications. In this section, we will explore practical tips and techniques for effectively managing dysphagia on a day-to-day basis.

1. Modify Food Consistency: Adjusting the texture of foods can make swallowing easier and safer. Depending on the individual's specific needs, foods may need to be pureed, minced, or mashed. This helps ensure a smoother passage through the throat and reduces the risk of choking or aspiration. Consultation with a speech-language pathologist or a dietitian can provide guidance on appropriate food textures.

2. Optimal Food Preparation: Pay attention to the preparation of meals to enhance swallowability. It's important to cook foods until they are soft and tender, making them easier to chew and swallow. Cutting food into small, bite-sized pieces and avoiding tough or hard-to-chew items can also aid in safe swallowing.

3. Proper Eating Techniques: Adopting specific eating techniques can support better swallowing. Take smaller bites and chew food thoroughly before swallowing. Avoid rushing through meals and ensure a relaxed and upright sitting position while eating. Minimize distractions during meals to focus on the eating process and facilitate safe swallowing.

4. Adequate Liquid Consistency: Adjusting the consistency of liquids may be necessary for individuals with dysphagia. Thickening agents can be used to modify the viscosity of liquids, making them easier to control and reducing the risk of aspiration. However, it is crucial to follow the recommendations of healthcare professionals regarding the appropriate thickness for liquids.

5. Stay Hydrated: Adequate hydration is essential for overall health, including maintaining proper swallowing function. If thin liquids are a challenge, consider sipping on thickened liquids, consuming foods with high water content (e.g., soups, fruits), or using strategies such as swallowing multiple small sips instead of large gulps.

6. Mealtime Environment: Create a supportive environment during meals. Minimize distractions, such as loud noises or excessive conversation, which can interfere with focus and swallowing. Sit in an upright position,

preferably at a table, and maintain good posture to facilitate the swallowing process.

7. Assistive Devices: Various assistive devices can aid in managing dysphagia. Specialized eating utensils, such as angled spoons or cups with spouts, can make self-feeding easier. Additionally, using straws, particularly with one-way valves or anti-aspiration features, can help control liquid flow and reduce the risk of aspiration.

8. Communication and Education: Inform family members, friends, and caregivers about your dysphagia condition so that they can provide appropriate support. Educating those around you about the signs of choking and how to respond in an emergency can be vital. Effective communication can help create a safe and understanding environment.

9. Follow Medical Recommendations: It is crucial to adhere to the advice and recommendations of healthcare professionals involved in managing your dysphagia. This may include attending therapy sessions with a speech-language pathologist, taking prescribed medications, or undergoing any necessary medical procedures.

10. Emotional Support: Coping with dysphagia can sometimes be emotionally challenging. Seek support from support groups, online communities, or counseling services to connect with others facing similar experiences and to address any emotional or psychological aspects of living with dysphagia.

Working with Your Healthcare Team

When managing a condition like dysphagia, establishing a collaborative relationship with your healthcare team is crucial. A multidisciplinary approach involving various professionals can provide comprehensive care and support tailored to your specific needs. In this section, we will explore the importance of working with your healthcare team and offer guidance on how to effectively collaborate with them.

1. Identify Relevant Healthcare Professionals: Start by identifying the key healthcare professionals who can assist you in managing dysphagia. This may include a speech-language pathologist specializing in swallowing disorders, a gastroenterologist, a dietitian, and potentially other specialists depending on the underlying cause of your dysphagia. Your primary care physician can guide you in finding the appropriate specialists.

2. Open and Honest Communication: Establishing open and honest communication with your healthcare team is paramount. Share your symptoms, concerns, and any changes in your condition with them. Be proactive in discussing your goals, expectations, and preferences for treatment. Effective communication helps your healthcare providers better understand your needs and tailor their approach accordingly.

3. Active Participation: Take an active role in your healthcare journey. Educate yourself about dysphagia, its causes, and available treatment options. Ask questions to clarify any uncertainties and seek explanations for medical terminologies or procedures. This active participation empowers you to make informed decisions and actively contribute to your own care.

4. Follow Treatment Plans: Adherence to treatment plans is crucial for effective management of dysphagia. Follow the instructions provided by your healthcare team regarding dietary modifications, medication regimens, therapy exercises, and any other recommended interventions. Consistency and compliance with the prescribed treatment plan can lead to better outcomes.

5. Regular Check-ups and Monitoring: Schedule regular appointments with your healthcare providers to monitor your progress and address any concerns that may arise. These check-ups allow your healthcare team to assess your condition, make adjustments to your treatment plan if necessary, and provide ongoing support and guidance.

6. Collaborative Goal Setting: Work with your healthcare team to establish realistic and attainable goals. This could include improving swallowing function, reducing symptoms, maintaining or gaining weight, or enhancing overall quality of life. Collaboratively setting goals ensures that everyone is aligned and working towards a shared objective.

7. Integrated Care: Encourage coordination and communication among your healthcare providers. Your speech-language pathologist, gastroenterologist, and dietitian, for example, should work together to develop a holistic approach to managing dysphagia. Be proactive in facilitating this integrated care by sharing relevant information and updates between your healthcare team members.

8. Seek Second Opinions if Needed: If you have concerns about your diagnosis or treatment plan, it is perfectly acceptable to seek a second opinion. Another healthcare professional with expertise in dysphagia can provide a fresh perspective and offer alternative recommendations. Remember, it's your health, and you have the right to explore different options.

9. Emotional Support: Dealing with dysphagia can be emotionally challenging. Your healthcare team can provide guidance and support, but don't hesitate to seek additional emotional support if needed. Support groups, counseling services, or online communities can offer valuable insights, advice, and a sense of camaraderie with others facing similar challenges.

10. Long-Term Management: Dysphagia may require long-term management, and your healthcare team will play a vital role in this process. Stay engaged with your providers, attend follow-up appointments, and communicate any changes or concerns promptly. Regular monitoring and ongoing collaboration with your healthcare team can help ensure that your management plan evolves as needed.

Modified food textures and thickened liquids are common interventions used in the management of dysphagia. These modifications help individuals with swallowing difficulties safely consume food and liquids, reduce the risk of choking or aspiration, and enhance overall swallowing function. Let's explore modified food textures and thickened liquids in more detail:

Modified Food Textures:

1. Pureed: Foods are blended to a smooth, cohesive texture without any lumps or solid pieces. Pureed foods are often used for individuals with severe swallowing difficulties or who have challenges chewing and managing larger food particles.

2. Minced: Foods are finely chopped into small, easily manageable pieces. The texture is softer and less cohesive than pureed foods, allowing individuals to control the bolus more effectively during swallowing.

3. Mashed: Foods are mashed or mashed with liquids to create a soft and cohesive texture. Mashed foods maintain some texture and may contain small soft lumps, making them suitable for individuals with moderate swallowing difficulties.

4. Soft: Foods that are naturally soft or cooked until they reach a tender consistency. Soft-textured foods are easier to chew and swallow, making them more manageable for individuals with mild swallowing difficulties.

The specific texture modifications needed will depend on an individual's swallowing abilities and recommendations from their healthcare team. Speech-language pathologists and dietitians often play a significant role in determining appropriate food textures based on individual needs and swallowing assessments.

Thickened Liquids:

Thickening liquids is another strategy used to manage dysphagia. Thickened liquids help control the flow and reduce the risk of aspiration. The consistency of thickened liquids is adjusted based on an individual's swallowing abilities and recommendations from healthcare professionals. Common thickening agents include:

1. Thickening Powders: Commercially available powders, such as modified food starch or xanthan gum, can be added to liquids to increase their viscosity. These powders come in different thickness levels, ranging from nectar-thick to honey-thick to pudding-thick.

2. Thickening Gels: Some thickening agents are in gel form, which can be mixed with liquids to achieve the desired consistency. These gels are often pre-measured and come in individual packets for convenience.

It is important to follow the specific instructions provided by healthcare professionals regarding the appropriate thickness level for liquids. Using the correct consistency helps ensure safe swallowing and reduce the risk of aspiration pneumonia.

It's worth noting that while modified food textures and thickened liquids can improve safety during swallowing, they may impact the sensory experience of eating and drinking. Working with a speech-language pathologist and dietitian can help find a balance between safety and maintaining enjoyment and nutritional intake.

Remember, individual needs may vary, and it's essential to consult with healthcare professionals to determine the most appropriate modified food textures and thickened liquids for your specific condition and swallowing abilities.

Essential Kitchen Tools for Dysphagia Cooking

When managing dysphagia, having the right kitchen tools can make meal preparation easier and ensure that modified foods are prepared safely and efficiently. Here are some essential kitchen tools that can be helpful when cooking for dysphagia:

1. Blender or Food Processor: A high-quality blender or food processor is essential for creating pureed or minced textures. These appliances can effectively blend or chop foods into smooth or finely chopped consistencies, making them easier to swallow.

2. Strainer or Sieve: A fine-mesh strainer or sieve can be used to remove any lumps or solid particles from pureed foods, ensuring a smoother texture. This is particularly helpful when preparing pureed soups, sauces, or fruits.

3. Food Mill: A food mill is a manual kitchen tool that can be used to puree or strain cooked foods. It helps remove skins, seeds, and fibrous parts from fruits and vegetables, resulting in a smooth and uniform texture.

4. Immersion Blender: An immersion blender, also known as a hand blender, is a versatile tool that can be used directly in pots or containers to blend soups, sauces, or other cooked foods. It eliminates the need to transfer hot liquids to a separate blender.

5. Chopper or Food Chopper: A chopper or food chopper can be useful for mincing or finely chopping foods. It can make the process quicker and more efficient, especially when preparing minced textures for recipes.

6. Food Scale: A food scale helps in accurately measuring ingredients, especially when following specific recipes or dietary guidelines. It ensures precise measurements for modified food preparation and portion control.

7. Measuring Cups and Spoons: Having a set of measuring cups and spoons is essential for accurate portioning and measuring of ingredients. This is particularly important when following modified recipes or dietary recommendations.

8. Non-Slip Cutting Board: A non-slip cutting board provides stability and prevents it from sliding during food preparation. Look for a cutting board

with rubberized grips or non-slip feet to ensure safety while cutting or chopping ingredients.

9. Adaptive Utensils: Adaptive utensils, such as angled spoons or utensils with built-up handles, can be helpful for individuals with limited dexterity or motor control. These utensils make self-feeding easier and more comfortable.

10. Thickening Agent Measuring Cups: If you regularly prepare thickened liquids, having measuring cups specifically designed for thickening agents can help ensure accurate and consistent measurements. These cups are labeled with thickened liquid levels (e.g., nectar-thick, honey-thick) for convenience.

Remember to clean and maintain these kitchen tools properly to ensure food safety and hygiene. Additionally, consult with a speech-language pathologist or dietitian for specific recommendations on modified food preparation and suitable kitchen tools based on your individual needs.

Having the right kitchen tools can simplify the process of preparing modified foods for dysphagia, making mealtime safer and more enjoyable.

Chapter 2:

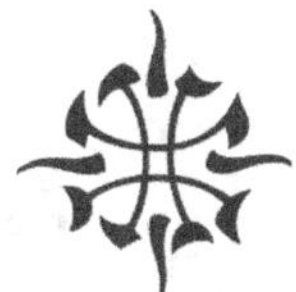

SMOOTH PUREES

Creamy Butternut Squash Soup:

- Preparation Time: 15 minutes

- Cooking Time: 40 minutes

- Servings: 4

Ingredients:

- 1 butternut squash, peeled, seeded, and cubed

- 1 onion, chopped

- 2 cloves of garlic, minced

- 1 tablespoon olive oil

- 4 cups vegetable or chicken broth

- 1/2 teaspoon ground cinnamon

- 1/4 teaspoon ground nutmeg

- Salt and pepper to taste

- Optional toppings: a drizzle of cream, roasted pumpkin seeds, or chopped fresh herbs

Directions:

1. Heat the olive oil in a large pot over medium heat. Add the chopped onion and minced garlic, and sauté until they become translucent and fragrant.

2. Add the cubed butternut squash, cinnamon, nutmeg, salt, and pepper to the pot. Stir well to coat the squash with the spices.

3. Pour in the vegetable or chicken broth, ensuring that the squash is fully covered. Bring the mixture to a boil, then reduce the heat to low, cover the pot, and simmer for about 30 minutes or until the squash is tender.

4. Use an immersion blender or transfer the mixture to a blender in batches to puree the soup until smooth and creamy.

5. Return the soup to the pot and heat over low heat for a few more minutes, stirring occasionally. Adjust the seasoning as needed.

6. Serve the creamy butternut squash soup hot, garnished with a drizzle of cream, roasted pumpkin seeds, or chopped fresh herbs if desired.

Nutrition: (per serving - without toppings)

- Calories: 150

- Fat: 4g

- Carbohydrates: 30g

- Fiber: 6g

- Protein: 3g

Silky Carrot Ginger Puree:

- Preparation Time: 10 minutes

- Cooking Time: 25 minutes

- Servings: 4

Ingredients:

- 1 pound carrots, peeled and chopped

- 1 small onion, chopped

- 2 cloves of garlic, minced

- 1 tablespoon fresh ginger, grated

- 4 cups vegetable broth

- 1 tablespoon olive oil

- Salt and pepper to taste

- Optional toppings: a dollop of Greek yogurt, chopped fresh herbs, or toasted sesame seeds

Directions:

1. In a large pot, heat the olive oil over medium heat. Add the chopped onion, minced garlic, and grated ginger. Sauté until the onion becomes translucent and fragrant.

2. Add the chopped carrots to the pot and stir well to combine with the onion mixture.

3. Pour in the vegetable broth, ensuring that the carrots are fully covered. Bring the mixture to a boil, then reduce the heat to low, cover the pot, and simmer for about 20-25 minutes or until the carrots are tender.

4. Use an immersion blender or transfer the mixture to a blender in batches to puree the soup until silky smooth.

5. Return the pureed soup to the pot and heat over low heat for a few more minutes, stirring occasionally. Season with salt and pepper to taste.

6. Serve the silky carrot ginger puree hot, garnished with a dollop of Greek yogurt, chopped fresh herbs, or toasted sesame seeds if desired.

Nutrition: (per serving - without toppings)

- Calories: 110

- Fat: 3g

- Carbohydrates: 20g

- Fiber: 5g

- Protein: 2g

Velvety Potato Leek Soup:

- Preparation Time: 15 minutes

- Cooking Time: 30 minutes

- Servings: 4

Ingredients:

- 4 medium-sized potatoes, peeled and diced

- 2 leeks, white and light green parts only, sliced

- 2 cloves of garlic, minced

- 4 cups vegetable or chicken broth

- 1 tablespoon butter

- 1/2 cup heavy cream

- Salt and pepper to taste

- Optional toppings: chopped chives, crispy bacon bits, or grated cheese

Directions:

1. In a large pot, melt the butter over medium heat. Add the sliced leeks and minced garlic, and sauté until they become soft and fragrant.

2. Add the diced potatoes to the pot and stir well to combine with the leeks and garlic.

3. Pour in the vegetable or chicken broth, ensuring that the potatoes are fully covered. Bring the mixture to a boil, then reduce the heat to low, cover the pot, and simmer for about 20-25 minutes or until the potatoes are tender.

4. Use an immersion blender or transfer the mixture to a blender in batches to puree the soup until velvety smooth.

5. Return the pureed soup to the pot and stir in the heavy cream. Heat over low heat for a few more minutes, stirring occasionally. Season with salt and pepper totaste.

6. Serve the velvety potato leek soup hot, garnished with chopped chives, crispy bacon bits, or grated cheese if desired.

Nutrition: (per serving - without toppings)

- Calories: 250

- Fat: 14g

- Carbohydrates: 28g

- Fiber: 3g

- Protein: 4g

Smooth Spinach and Feta Puree:

- Preparation Time: 10 minutes

- Cooking Time: 10 minutes

- Servings: 4

Ingredients:

- 8 ounces fresh spinach leaves

- 1/2 cup crumbled feta cheese

- 2 cloves of garlic, minced

- 1 tablespoon olive oil

- 1/4 teaspoon dried oregano

- Salt and pepper to taste

Directions:

1. Heat the olive oil in a large skillet over medium heat. Add the minced garlic and sauté until fragrant.

2. Add the spinach leaves to the skillet and cook until wilted, stirring occasionally. This should take about 3-5 minutes.

3. Remove the skillet from heat and let the spinach cool slightly.

4. Place the cooked spinach, crumbled feta cheese, dried oregano, salt, and pepper in a blender or food processor and blend until smooth and creamy.

5. Adjust the seasoning if needed.

6. Serve the smooth spinach and feta puree warm or at room temperature.

Nutrition: (per serving)

- Calories: 120

- Fat: 9g

- Carbohydrates: 5g

- Fiber: 2g

- Protein: 6g

Creamy Cauliflower Mash:

- Preparation Time: 10 minutes

- Cooking Time: 20 minutes

- Servings: 4

Ingredients:

- 1 large head of cauliflower, cut into florets

- 2 cloves of garlic, minced

- 2 tablespoons butter

- 1/4 cup heavy cream

- Salt and pepper to taste

- Optional toppings: chopped fresh herbs or grated Parmesan cheese

Directions:

1. Steam or boil the cauliflower florets until they are very tender. This should take about 10-15 minutes.

2. In a small saucepan, melt the butter over low heat. Add the minced garlic and cook until fragrant, stirring occasionally.

3. Drain the cooked cauliflower and transfer it to a large bowl.

4. Pour the melted butter and garlic mixture over the cauliflower. Add the heavy cream.

5. Use a potato masher or an immersion blender to mash or blend the cauliflower until creamy and smooth. If needed, add more cream for desired consistency.

6. Season with salt and pepper to taste.

7. Serve the creamy cauliflower mash hot, garnished with chopped fresh herbs or grated Parmesan cheese if desired.

Nutrition: (per serving - without toppings)

- Calories: 120

- Fat: 10g

- Carbohydrates: 6g

- Fiber: 3g

- Protein: 3g

Please note that the nutrition information provided is approximate and may vary based on specific ingredients and serving sizes.

- Preparation Time: 15 minutes

- Cooking Time: 40 minutes

- Servings: 4

Ingredients:

- 2 red bell peppers

- 4 medium-sized tomatoes

- 1 onion, chopped

- 2 cloves of garlic, minced

- 2 tablespoons olive oil

- 4 cups vegetable or chicken broth

- 1/2 cup heavy cream

- Salt and pepper to taste

- Optional toppings: a dollop of sour cream or Greek yogurt, freshly chopped basil or parsley

Directions:

1. Preheat the oven to 400°F (200°C).

2. Cut the red bell peppers in half and remove the seeds and stems. Place them on a baking sheet along with the whole tomatoes. Drizzle with olive oil and sprinkle with salt and pepper.

3. Roast the peppers and tomatoes in the preheated oven for about 25-30 minutes or until the skins are charred and blistered.

4. Remove the baking sheet from the oven and let the peppers and tomatoes cool slightly. Peel off the skins from the peppers and tomatoes.

5. In a large pot, heat the olive oil over medium heat. Add the chopped onion and minced garlic, and sauté until they become translucent and fragrant.

6. Add the roasted peppers and tomatoes to the pot, along with the vegetable or chicken broth. Bring the mixture to a boil, then reduce the heat to low, cover the pot, and simmer for about 15 minutes to allow the flavors to meld.

7. Use an immersion blender or transfer the mixture to a blender in batches to puree the soup until smooth.

8. Return the pureed soup to the pot and stir in the heavy cream. Heat over low heat for a few more minutes, stirring occasionally. Season with salt and pepper to taste.

9. Serve the roasted red pepper and tomato bisque hot, garnished with a dollop of sour cream or Greek yogurt, and freshly chopped basil or parsley if desired.

Nutrition: (per serving - without toppings)

- Calories: 180

- Fat: 13g

- Carbohydrates: 15g

- Fiber: 3g

- Protein: 4g

Broccoli and Cheddar Puree:

- Preparation Time: 10 minutes

- Cooking Time: 15 minutes

- Servings: 4

Ingredients:

- 2 cups broccoli florets

- 1 small onion, chopped

- 2 cloves of garlic, minced

- 2 tablespoons butter

- 2 cups vegetable or chicken broth

- 1 cup shredded cheddar cheese

- Salt and pepper to taste

Directions:

1. In a medium-sized pot, melt the butter over medium heat. Add the chopped onion and minced garlic, and sauté until they become translucent and fragrant.

2. Add the broccoli florets to the pot, along with the vegetable or chicken broth. Bring the mixture to a boil, then reduce the heat to low, cover the pot, and simmer for about 10-12 minutes or until the broccoli is tender.

3. Use an immersion blender or transfer the mixture to a blender in batches to puree the soup until smooth.

4. Return the pureed soup to the pot and stir in the shredded cheddar cheese. Heat over low heat until the cheese is melted and incorporated into the soup.

5. Season with salt and pepper to taste.

6. Serve the broccoli and cheddar puree hot.

Nutrition: (per serving)

- Calories: 200

- Fat: 15g

- Carbohydrates: 8g

- Fiber: 2g

- Protein: 9g

Comforting Cream of Mushroom Soup:

- Preparation Time: 10 minutes

- Cooking Time: 25 minutes

- Servings: 4

Ingredients:

- 16 ounces mushrooms, sliced

- 1 onion, chopped

- 2 cloves of garlic, minced

- 2 tablespoons butter

- 4 cups vegetable or chicken broth

- 1 cup heavy cream

- 2 tablespoons all-purpose flour (optional, for thickening)

- Salt and pepper to taste

- Optional toppings: sautéed mushrooms, chopped fresh parsley

Directions:

1. In a large pot, melt the butter over medium heat. Add the chopped onion and minced garlic, and sauté until they become translucent and fragrant.

2. Add the sliced mushrooms to the pot and cook until they release their moisture and become tender, stirring occasionally. This should take about 8-10 minutes.

3. Pour in the vegetable or chicken broth and bring the mixture to a simmer. Let it simmer for about 10 minutes to allow the flavors to develop.

4. Use an immersion blender or transfer the mixture to a blender in batches to puree the soup until smooth. If you prefer a chunkier texture, you can skip this step and leave some mushroom pieces.

5. Return the pureed soup to the pot and stir in the heavy cream. If you prefer a thicker consistency, you can mix 2 tablespoons of all-purpose flour with a little water to make a slurry and add it to the soup. Cook for an additional 5 minutes, stirring continuously, until the soup thickens.

6. Season with salt and pepper to taste.

7. Serve the comforting cream of mushroom soup hot, garnished with sautéed mushrooms and chopped fresh parsley if desired.

Nutrition: (per serving - without toppings)

- Calories: 240

- Fat: 20g

- Carbohydrates: 11g

- Fiber: 2g

- Protein: 5g

Creamy Asparagus and Parmesan Puree:

- Preparation Time: 10 minutes

- Cooking Time: 20 minutes

- Servings: 4

Ingredients:

- 1 bunch asparagus, ends trimmed and cut into 1-inch pieces

- 1 small onion, chopped

- 2 cloves of garlic, minced

- 2 tablespoons butter

- 4 cups vegetable or chicken broth

- 1/2 cup grated Parmesan cheese

- 1/4 cup heavy cream

- Salt and pepper to taste

Directions:

1. In a medium-sized pot, melt the butter over medium heat. Add the chopped onion and minced garlic, and sauté until they become translucent and fragrant.

2. Add the asparagus pieces to the pot and sauté for about 5 minutes until they are slightly tender.

3. Pour in the vegetable or chicken broth and bring the mixture to a simmer. Let it simmer for about 10-12 minutes or until the asparagus is fully cooked and tender.

4. Use an immersion blender or transfer the mixture to a blender in batches to puree the soup until smooth.

5. Return the pureed soup to the pot and stir in the grated Parmesan cheese and heavy cream. Heat over low heat until the cheese is melted and incorporated into the soup.

6. Season with salt and pepper to taste.

7. Serve the creamy asparagus and Parmesan puree hot.

Nutrition: (per serving)

- Calories: 180

- Fat: 13g

- Carbohydrates: 8g

- Fiber: 3g

- Protein: 8g

Sweet and Savory Pumpkin Puree:

- Preparation Time: 10 minutes

- Cooking Time: 25 minutes

- Servings: 4

Ingredients:

- 2 cups pumpkin puree (canned or homemade)

- 1 small onion, chopped

- 2 cloves of garlic, minced

- 2 tablespoons butter

- 4 cups vegetable or chicken broth

- 1/2 cup coconut milk (or heavy cream)

- 1 tablespoon maple syrup (optional, for sweetness)

- 1/2 teaspoon ground cinnamon

- 1/4 teaspoon ground nutmeg

- Salt and pepper to taste

- Optional toppings: roasted pumpkin seeds, a drizzle of coconut milk, chopped fresh chives

Directions:

1. In a large pot, melt the butter over medium heat. Add the chopped onion and minced garlic, and sauté until they become translucent and fragrant.

2. Add the pumpkin puree to the pot and stir well to combine with the onion and garlic.

3. Pour in the vegetable or chicken broth and bring the mixture to a simmer. Let it simmer for about 10-12 minutes to allow the flavors to develop.

4. Stir in the coconut milk (or heavy cream), maple syrup (if using), ground cinnamon, and ground nutmeg. Continue to cook for another 5 minutes.

5. Season with salt and pepper to taste.

6. Serve the sweet and savory pumpkin puree hot, garnished with roasted pumpkin seeds, a drizzle of coconut milk, and chopped fresh chives if desired.

Nutrition: (per serving - without toppings)

- Calories: 180

- Fat: 11g

- Carbohydrates: 19g

- Fiber: 4g

- Protein: 4g

Creamy Spinach and Ricotta Puree:

- Preparation Time: 10 minutes

- Cooking Time: 15 minutes

- Servings: 4

Ingredients:

- 1 pound fresh spinach leaves

- 1 small onion, chopped

- 2 cloves of garlic, minced

- 2 tablespoons olive oil

- 1 cup ricotta cheese

- 4 cups vegetable or chicken broth

- Salt and pepper to taste

- Optional toppings: grated Parmesan cheese, a drizzle of olive oil

Directions:

1. In a large pot, heat the olive oil over medium heat. Add the chopped onion and minced garlic, and sauté until they become translucent and fragrant.

2. Add the fresh spinach leaves to the pot and cook until wilted, stirring occasionally. This should take about 5 minutes.

3. Pour in the vegetable or chicken broth and bring the mixture to a simmer. Let it simmer for about 5-7 minutes to allow the flavors to meld.

4. Use an immersion blender or transfer the mixture to a blender in batches to puree the soup until smooth.

5. Return the pureed soup to the pot and stir in the ricotta cheese. Heat over low heat until the cheese is melted and incorporated into the soup.

6. Season with salt and pepper to taste.

7. Serve the creamy spinach and ricotta puree hot, garnished with grated Parmesan cheese and a drizzle of olive oil if desired.

Nutrition: (per serving - without toppings)

- Calories: 220

- Fat: 16g

- Carbohydrates: 10g

- Fiber: 3g

- Protein: 12g

Creamy Sweet Potato Puree:

- Preparation Time: 10 minutes

- Cooking Time: 25 minutes

- Servings: 4

Ingredients:

- 2 large sweet potatoes, peeled and cubed

- 1 small onion, chopped

- 2 cloves of garlic, minced

- 2 tablespoons butter

- 4 cups vegetable or chicken broth

- 1/2 cup coconut milk (or heavy cream)

- 1/2 teaspoon ground cinnamon

- 1/4 teaspoon ground nutmeg

- Salt and pepper to taste

- Optional toppings: toasted pecans, a sprinkle of cinnamon

Directions:

1. In a medium-sized pot, melt the butter over medium heat. Add the chopped onion and minced garlic, and sauté until they become translucent and fragrant.

2. Add the cubed sweet potatoes to the pot and cook for about 5 minutes, stirring occasionally.

3. Pour in the vegetable or chicken broth and bring the mixture to a simmer. Let it simmer for about 15-20 minutes or until the sweet potatoes are fork-tender.

4. Use an immersion blender or transfer the mixture to a blender in batches to puree the soup until smooth.

5. Return the pureed soup to the pot and stir in the coconut milk (or heavy cream), ground cinnamon, and ground nutmeg. Heat over low heat for a few more minutes, stirring occasionally.

6. Season with salt and pepper to taste.

7. Serve the creamy sweet potato puree hot, garnished with toasted pecans and a sprinkle of cinnamon if desired.

Nutrition: (per serving - without toppings)

- Calories: 250

- Fat: 12g

- Carbohydrates: 33g

- Fiber: 5g

- Protein: 4g

Smooth Pea and Mint Soup:

- Preparation Time: 10 minutes

- Cooking Time: 15 minutes

- Servings: 4

Ingredients:

- 2 cups frozen peas

- 1 small onion, chopped

- 2 cloves of garlic, minced

- 2 tablespoons butter

- 4 cups vegetable or chicken broth

- 1/4 cup fresh mint leaves

- 1/4 cup heavy cream

- Salt and pepper to taste

- Optional toppings: a dollop of Greek yogurt, freshly chopped mint

Directions:

1. In a large pot, melt the butter over medium heat. Add the chopped onion and minced garlic, and sauté until they become translucent and fragrant.

2. Add the frozen peas to the pot and cook for about 2-3 minutes until they are heated through.

3. Pour in the vegetable or chicken broth and bring the mixture to a simmer. Let it simmer for about 5-7 minutes to allow the flavors to meld.

4. Add the fresh mint leaves to the pot and stir well.

5. Use an immersion blender or transfer the mixture to a blender in batches to puree the soup until smooth.

6. Return the pureed soup to the pot and stir in the heavy cream. Heat over low heat for a few more minutes, stirring occasionally.

7. Season with salt and pepper to taste.

8. Serve the smooth pea and mint soup hot, garnished with a dollop ofGreek yogurt and freshly chopped mint if desired.

Nutrition: (per serving - without toppings)

- Calories: 180

- Fat: 10g

- Carbohydrates: 18g

- Fiber: 5g

- Protein: 6g

Creamy Avocado and Cucumber Puree:

- Preparation Time: 10 minutes

- Cooking Time: 0 minutes

- Servings: 4

Ingredients:

- 2 ripe avocados, pitted and peeled

- 1 large cucumber, peeled and chopped

- 1/4 cup fresh cilantro leaves

- 2 tablespoons lime juice

- 1 cup vegetable or chicken broth

- Salt and pepper to taste

- Optional toppings: diced cucumber, chopped cilantro

Directions:

1. In a blender or food processor, combine the ripe avocados, chopped cucumber, fresh cilantro leaves, lime juice, and vegetable or chicken broth.

2. Blend until smooth and creamy.

3. Season with salt and pepper to taste.

4. Serve the creamy avocado and cucumber puree chilled or at room temperature.

5. Garnish with diced cucumber and chopped cilantro if desired.

Nutrition: (per serving - without toppings)

- Calories: 200

- Fat: 16g

- Carbohydrates: 14g

- Fiber: 9g

- Protein: 4g

Creamy Zucchini and Basil Soup:

- Preparation Time: 10 minutes

- Cooking Time: 20 minutes

- Servings: 4

Ingredients:

- 2 medium zucchinis, chopped

- 1 small onion, chopped

- 2 cloves of garlic, minced

- 2 tablespoons olive oil

- 4 cups vegetable or chicken broth

- 1/2 cup fresh basil leaves

- 1/2 cup heavy cream

- Salt and pepper to taste

- Optional toppings: a drizzle of olive oil, fresh basil leaves

Directions:

1. In a large pot, heat the olive oil over medium heat. Add the chopped onion and minced garlic, and sauté until they become translucent and fragrant.

2. Add the chopped zucchinis to the pot and cook for about 5 minutes until they are slightly softened.

3. Pour in the vegetable or chicken broth and bring the mixture to a simmer. Let it simmer for about 10-15 minutes or until the zucchinis are tender.

4. Add the fresh basil leaves to the pot and stir well.

5. Use an immersion blender or transfer the mixture to a blender in batches to puree the soup until smooth.

6. Return the pureed soup to the pot and stir in the heavy cream. Heat over low heat for a few more minutes, stirring occasionally.

7. Season with salt and pepper to taste.

8. Serve the creamy zucchini and basil soup hot, garnished with a drizzle of olive oil and fresh basil leaves if desired.

Nutrition: (per serving - without toppings)

- Calories: 220

- Fat: 18g

- Carbohydrates: 10g

- Fiber: 2g

- Protein: 4g

Roasted Garlic and White Bean Puree:

- Preparation Time: 10 minutes

- Cooking Time: 45 minutes

- Servings: 4

Ingredients:

- 1 whole head of garlic

- 2 tablespoons olive oil

- 1 can (15 ounces) white beans, drained and rinsed

- 2 tablespoons lemon juice

- 1/4 cup fresh parsley, chopped

- Salt and pepper to taste

- Optional toppings: drizzle of olive oil, chopped parsley

Directions:

1. Preheat the oven to 400°F (200°C).

2. Cut off the top of the head of garlic to expose the cloves. Place the garlic on a piece of aluminum foil and drizzle with olive oil. Wrap the garlic tightly in the foil.

3. Roast the garlic in the preheated oven for about 30-40 minutes or until the cloves are soft and golden.

4. Allow the roasted garlic to cool slightly, then squeeze the cloves out of their skins into a blender or food processor.

5. Add the white beans, lemon juice, and fresh parsley to the blender or food processor. Blend until smooth and creamy.

6. Season the puree with salt and pepper to taste.

7. Serve the roasted garlic and white bean puree warm or at room temperature.

8. Garnish with a drizzle of olive oil and chopped parsley if desired.

Nutrition: (per serving - without toppings)

- Calories: 180

- Fat: 7g

- Carbohydrates: 24g

- Fiber: 6g

- Protein: 8g

Creamy Beetroot Puree:

- Preparation Time: 10 minutes

- Cooking Time: 35 minutes

- Servings: 4

Ingredients:

- 4 medium beetroots, peeled and chopped

- 1 small onion, chopped

- 2 cloves of garlic, minced

- 2 tablespoons butter

- 4 cups vegetable or chicken broth

- 1/4 cup sour cream

- Salt and pepper to taste

- Optional toppings: dollop of sour cream, fresh dill

Directions:

1. In a large pot, melt the butter over medium heat. Add the chopped onion and minced garlic, and sauté until they become translucent and fragrant.

2. Add the chopped beetroots to the pot and cook for about 5 minutes, stirring occasionally.

3. Pour in the vegetable or chicken broth and bring the mixture to a simmer. Let it simmer for about 25-30 minutes or until the beetroots are fork-tender.

4. Use an immersion blender or transfer the mixture to a blender in batches to puree the soup until smooth.

5. Return the pureed soup to the pot and stir in the sour cream. Heat over low heat for a few more minutes, stirring occasionally.

6. Season with salt and pepper to taste.

7. Serve the creamy beetroot puree hot, garnished with a dollop of sour cream and fresh dill if desired.

Nutrition: (per serving - without toppings)

- Calories: 160

- Fat: 8g

- Carbohydrates: 20g

- Fiber: 5g

- Protein: 4g

- Preparation Time: 10 minutes

- Cooking Time: 40 minutes

- Servings: 4

Ingredients:

- 1 cup red lentils

- 1 small onion, chopped

- 2 cloves of garlic, minced

- 1 tablespoon olive oil

- 1 teaspoon ground cumin

- 1 teaspoon ground coriander

- 1/2 teaspoon ground turmeric

- 4 cups vegetable or chicken broth

- 1/4 cup coconut milk (optional)

- Salt and pepper to taste

- Optional toppings: chopped cilantro, a squeeze of lemon juice

Directions:

1. Rinse the red lentils under cold water until the water runs clear.

2. In a large pot, heat the olive oil over medium heat. Add the chopped onion and minced garlic, and sauté until they become translucent and fragrant.

3. Add the rinsed lentils, ground cumin, ground coriander, and ground turmeric to the pot. Stir well to coat the lentils with the spices.

4. Pour in the vegetable or chicken broth and bring the mixture to a boil. Reduce the heat and let it simmer for about 30 minutes or until the lentils are soft and tender.

5. Use an immersion blender or transfer the mixture to a blender in batches to puree the soup until smooth.

6. Return the pureed soup to the pot and stir in the coconut milk if desired. Heat over low heat for a few more minutes, stirring occasionally.

7. Season with salt and pepper to taste.

8. Serve the smooth lentil dal hot, garnished with chopped cilantro and a squeeze of lemon juice if desired

Creamy Chicken and Vegetable Puree:

- Preparation Time: 15 minutes

- Cooking Time: 25 minutes

- Servings: 4

Ingredients:

- 2 boneless, skinless chicken breasts, cut into small pieces

- 1 tablespoon olive oil

- 1 small onion, chopped

- 2 cloves of garlic, minced

- 2 carrots, peeled and chopped

- 2 celery stalks, chopped

- 4 cups chicken broth

- 1 cup frozen peas

- 1/2 cup heavy cream

- Salt and pepper to taste

- Optional toppings: chopped parsley, grated Parmesan cheese

Directions:

1. In a large pot, heat the olive oil over medium heat. Add the chopped onion and minced garlic, and sauté until they become translucent and fragrant.

2. Add the chicken pieces to the pot and cook until they are browned on all sides.

3. Add the chopped carrots and celery to the pot and cook for a few minutes until they begin to soften.

4. Pour in the chicken broth and bring the mixture to a boil. Reduce the heat and let it simmer for about 15 minutes or until the chicken is cooked through and the vegetables are tender.

5. Stir in the frozen peas and cook for another 2-3 minutes until they are heated through.

6. Use an immersion blender or transfer the mixture to a blender in batches to puree the soup until smooth.

7. Return the pureed soup to the pot and stir in the heavy cream. Heat over low heat for a few more minutes, stirring occasionally.

8. Season with salt and pepper to taste.

9. Serve the creamy chicken and vegetable puree hot, garnished with chopped parsley and grated Parmesan cheese if desired.

Nutrition: (per serving - without toppings)

- Calories: 280

- Fat: 14g

- Carbohydrates: 16g

- Fiber: 3g

- Protein: 22g

Creamy Mango and Banana Puree:

- Preparation Time: 5 minutes

- Servings: 2

Ingredients:

- 1 ripe mango, peeled and diced

- 1 ripe banana, peeled and sliced

- 1/2 cup plain Greek yogurt

- 1 tablespoon honey (optional)

- 1/2 teaspoon vanilla extract (optional)

- Optional toppings: sliced mango, banana slices, shredded coconut

Directions:

1. Place the diced mango, sliced banana, Greek yogurt, honey (if using), and vanilla extract (if using) in a blender or food processor.

2. Blend the ingredients until smooth and creamy.

3. Taste and adjust the sweetness with more honey if desired.

4. Pour the creamy mango and banana puree into serving bowls.

5. Garnish with sliced mango, banana slices, and shredded coconut if desired.

6. Serve the puree chilled.

Nutrition: (per serving - without toppings)

- Calories: 180

- Fat: 1g

- Carbohydrates: 42g

- Fiber: 4g

- Protein: 9g

Chapter 3:

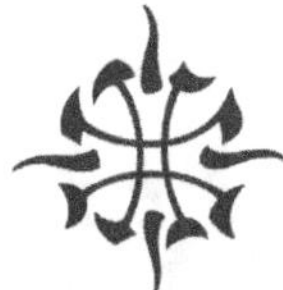

Soft and Tender Dishes

Tender Slow-Cooked Pot Roast

Preparation Time: 15 minutes

Cooking Time: 8 hours (slow cooker)

Servings:6

Ingredients:

- 3 lb beef chuck roast

- 1 tablespoon olive oil

- 1 onion, sliced

- 3 carrots, peeled and cut into chunks

- 3 potatoes, peeled and cut into chunks

- 2 cups beef broth

- 2 tablespoons tomato paste

- 2 teaspoons Worcestershire sauce

- 2 cloves garlic, minced

- 1 teaspoon dried thyme

- 1 teaspoon dried rosemary

- Salt and pepper to taste

Directions:

1. Season the roast with salt and pepper. In a large skillet, heat olive oil over medium-high heat and brown the roast on all sides.

2. Place the sliced onion, carrots, and potatoes in the bottom of a slow cooker. Put the browned roast on top.

3. In a bowl, mix together beef broth, tomato paste, Worcestershire sauce, garlic, thyme, and rosemary. Pour over the roast.

4. Cover and cook on low for 8 hours, or until the meat is tender and easily shredded.

5. Remove the roast and vegetables from the slow cooker. Let the meat rest for a few minutes before slicing. Serve with the cooked vegetables and gravy.

Nutrition (per serving):

- Calories: 400

- Protein: 35g

- Carbohydrates: 20g

- Fat: 20g

- Fiber: 3g

- Sodium: 600mg

Preparation Time: 5 minutes

Cooking Time: 5 minutes

Servings: 2

Ingredients:

- 4 large eggs

- 2 tablespoons milk or cream

- 1 tablespoon butter

- Salt and pepper to taste

- Fresh chives or parsley for garnish (optional)

Directions:

1. In a bowl, whisk together eggs, milk, salt, and pepper until well combined.

2. Heat a non-stick skillet over medium-low heat and add butter.

3. Pour the egg mixture into the skillet. Let it sit for a few seconds until the edges start to set.

4. Gently stir the eggs with a spatula, moving them from the edges to the center. Continue until the eggs are softly scrambled and slightly runny.

5. Remove from heat immediately to avoid overcooking. Garnish with fresh chives or parsley if desired, and serve warm.

Nutrition (per serving):

- Calories: 180

- Protein: 12g

- Carbohydrates: 1g

- Fat: 14g

- Fiber: 0g

- Sodium: 200mg

Moist and Tender Baked Salmon

Preparation Time:10 minutes

Cooking Time: 20 minutes

Servings: 4

 Ingredients:

- 4 salmon fillets

- 2 tablespoons olive oil

- 1 lemon, thinly sliced

- 2 cloves garlic, minced

- 1 teaspoon dried dill

- Salt and pepper to taste

Directions:

1. Preheat oven to 375°F (190°C). Line a baking sheet with parchment paper.

2. Place salmon fillets on the prepared baking sheet. Drizzle with olive oil and sprinkle with garlic, dill, salt, and pepper.

3. Top each fillet with lemon slices.

4. Bake for 15-20 minutes, or until the salmon flakes easily with a fork.

5. Serve immediately with your choice of side dishes.

Nutrition (per serving):

- Calories: 300

- Protein: 25g

- Carbohydrates: 1g

- Fat: 21g

- Fiber: 0g

- Sodium: 300mg

Tender Meatballs in Tomato Sauce

Preparation Time:20 minutes

Cooking Time: 30 minutes

Servings: 4

Ingredients:

- 1 lb ground beef

- 1/2 cup breadcrumbs

- 1/4 cup grated Parmesan cheese

- 1 egg

- 2 cloves garlic, minced

- 2 tablespoons fresh parsley, chopped

- 1 teaspoon salt

- 1/2 teaspoon black pepper

- 2 cups marinara sauce

- 1 tablespoon olive oil

Directions:

1. In a large bowl, combine ground beef, breadcrumbs, Parmesan cheese, egg, garlic, parsley, salt, and pepper. Mix until well combined.

2. Form the mixture into small meatballs (about 1 inch in diameter).

3. In a large skillet, heat olive oil over medium heat. Add the meatballs and cook until browned on all sides.

4. Pour marinara sauce over the meatballs. Reduce heat to low, cover, and simmer for 20-25 minutes until the meatballs are cooked through.

5. Serve meatballs with sauce over pasta or with a side of bread.

Nutrition (per serving):

- Calories: 350

- Protein: 20g

- Carbohydrates: 15g

- Fat: 22g

- Fiber: 3g

- Sodium: 800mg

Soft and Creamy Macaroni and Cheese

Preparation Time: 10 minutes

Cooking Time: 25 minutes

Servings: 4

Ingredients:

- 2 cups elbow macaroni

- 4 tablespoons butter

- 4 tablespoons all-purpose flour

- 2 cups milk

- 2 cups shredded cheddar cheese

- 1/2 teaspoon salt

- 1/4 teaspoon black pepper

- 1/4 teaspoon garlic powder (optional)

Directions:

1. Cook the macaroni according to package directions. Drain and set aside.

2. In a saucepan, melt butter over medium heat. Stir in flour and cook for 1-2 minutes until smooth and bubbly.

3. Gradually add milk, stirring constantly until the mixture thickens.

4. Add cheese, salt, pepper, and garlic powder. Stir until cheese is melted and the sauce is smooth.

5. Combine the cheese sauce with the cooked macaroni. Mix well and serve warm.

Nutrition (per serving):

- Calories: 450

- Protein: 16g

- Carbohydrates: 48g

- Fat: 21g

- Fiber: 2g

- Sodium: 610mg

Tender Chicken and Mushroom Risotto

Preparation Time: 15 minutes

Cooking Time:30 minutes

Servings: 4

Ingredients:

- 2 tablespoons olive oil

- 1 onion, finely chopped

- 2 garlic cloves, minced

- 1 cup Arborio rice

- 4 cups chicken broth, warmed

- 1 cup cooked chicken breast, diced

- 1 cup sliced mushrooms

- 1/2 cup grated Parmesan cheese

- 2 tablespoons butter

- Salt and pepper to taste

- Fresh parsley for garnish

Directions:

1. Heat olive oil in a large saucepan over medium heat. Add onion and garlic, and sauté until translucent.

2. Add Arborio rice and cook, stirring, for 2-3 minutes until lightly toasted.

3. Gradually add warm chicken broth, one ladle at a time, stirring continuously until each addition is absorbed before adding the next.

4. After about 20 minutes, add the chicken and mushrooms. Continue to cook until the rice is tender and creamy.

5. Stir in Parmesan cheese and butter. Season with salt and pepper.

6. Garnish with fresh parsley and serve.

Nutrition (per serving):

- Calories: 400

- Protein: 20g

- Carbohydrates: 50g

- Fat: 15g

- Fiber: 2g

- Sodium: 600mg

Easy-to-Swallow Meatloaf

Preparation Time: 15 minutes

Cooking Time:1 hour

Servings: 4

 Ingredients:

- 1 lb ground beef

- 1/2 cup breadcrumbs

- 1/2 cup milk

- 1 egg

- 1 small onion, finely chopped

- 2 cloves garlic, minced

- 1/4 cup ketchup

- 1 tablespoon Worcestershire sauce

- 1 teaspoon salt

- 1/2 teaspoon black pepper

- 1/4 cup grated Parmesan cheese (optional)

Directions:

1. Preheat oven to 350°F (175°C).

2. In a large bowl, combine all ingredients. Mix until well blended.

3. Shape the mixture into a loaf and place it in a baking dish.

4. Bake for 1 hour, or until the internal temperature reaches 160°F (71°C).

5. Let rest for 10 minutes before slicing and serving.

Nutrition (per serving):

- Calories: 350

- Protein: 20g

- Carbohydrates: 15g

- Fat: 22g

- Fiber: 1g

- Sodium: 750mg

Soft and Tender Baked Chicken Breast

Preparation Time: 10 minutes

Cooking Time: 25 minutes

Servings:4

Ingredients:

- 4 boneless, skinless chicken breasts

- 2 tablespoons olive oil

- 1 teaspoon garlic powder

- 1 teaspoon onion powder

- 1 teaspoon paprika

- 1/2 teaspoon salt

- 1/2 teaspoon black pepper

Directions:

1. Preheat oven to 375°F (190°C).

2. Place chicken breasts in a baking dish. Drizzle with olive oil.

3. In a small bowl, combine garlic powder, onion powder, paprika, salt, and pepper. Sprinkle over the chicken.

4. Cover the baking dish with foil and bake for 20-25 minutes, or until the chicken is cooked through (internal temperature of 165°F or 74°C).

5. Let rest for 5 minutes before serving.

Nutrition (per serving):

- Calories: 220

- Protein: 26g

- Carbohydrates: 1g

- Fat: 12g

- Fiber: 0g

- Sodium: 400mg

Preparation Time: 20 minutes

Cooking Time: 2 hours 30 minutes

Servings: 6

Ingredients:

- 2 lb beef chuck, cut into 1-inch cubes

- 3 tablespoons all-purpose flour

- 2 tablespoons olive oil

- 1 onion, chopped

- 3 cloves garlic, minced

- 4 cups beef broth

- 1 cup red wine (optional)

- 4 carrots, peeled and cut into chunks

- 4 potatoes, peeled and cut into chunks

- 2 celery stalks, sliced

- 2 tablespoons tomato paste

- 1 teaspoon dried thyme

- 1 bay leaf

- Salt and pepper to taste

- Fresh parsley for garnish

Directions:

1. Toss the beef cubes in flour until well coated.

2. Heat olive oil in a large pot over medium-high heat. Brown the beef on all sides, then remove and set aside.

3. In the same pot, add onion and garlic. Cook until softened.

4. Stir in beef broth, red wine (if using), tomato paste, thyme, bay leaf, salt, and pepper.

5. Return beef to the pot. Add carrots, potatoes, and celery.

6. Bring to a boil, then reduce heat to low. Cover and simmer for about 2 hours, or until the beef is tender.

7. Remove bay leaf, garnish with parsley, and serve.

Nutrition (per serving):

- Calories: 450

- Protein: 30g

- Carbohydrates: 30g

- Fat: 20g

- Fiber: 5g

- Sodium: 700mg

Moist and Flavorful Turkey Meatballs

Preparation Time: 15 minutes

Cooking Time: 25 minutes

Servings: 4

Ingredients:

- 1 lb ground turkey

- 1/2 cup breadcrumbs

- 1/4 cup grated Parmesan cheese

- 1 egg

- 2 cloves garlic, minced

- 2 tablespoons fresh parsley, chopped

- 1 teaspoon salt

- 1/2 teaspoon black pepper

- 1/2 teaspoon dried oregano

- 1 tablespoon olive oil

Directions:

1. Preheat oven to 375°F (190°C).

2. In a large bowl, combine ground turkey, breadcrumbs, Parmesan cheese, egg, garlic, parsley, salt, pepper, and oregano. Mix until well combined.

3. Form the mixture into small meatballs and place on a baking sheet lined with parchment paper.

4. Drizzle with olive oil and bake for 20-25 minutes, or until the meatballs are cooked through and golden brown.

5. Serve with your favorite sauce or over pasta.

Nutrition (per serving):

- Calories: 250

- Protein: 25g

- Carbohydrates: 10g

- Fat: 12g

- Fiber: 1g

- Sodium: 500mg

Soft and Creamy Mashed Potatoes

Preparation Time: 10 minutes

Cooking Time: 20 minutes

Servings: 4

Ingredients:

- 2 lb potatoes, peeled and cut into chunks

- 1/2 cup milk

- 1/4 cup butter

- Salt and pepper to taste

- Fresh chives for garnish (optional)

 Directions:

1. Place potatoes in a large pot and cover with cold water. Bring to a boil and cook until tender, about 15-20 minutes.

2. Drain the potatoes and return to the pot.

3. Add milk and butter. Mash until smooth and creamy.

4. Season with salt and pepper to taste.

5. Garnish with fresh chives if desired, and serve warm.

Nutrition (per serving):

- Calories: 200

- Protein: 4g

- Carbohydrates: 30g

- Fat: 8g

- Fiber: 3g

- Sodium: 150mg

Tender Baked Cod with Lemon Butter Sauce

Preparation Time: 10 minutes

Cooking Time: 20 minutes

Servings: 4

Ingredients:

- 4 cod fillets

- 1/4 cup butter, melted

- 1 lemon, juiced and zested

- 2 cloves garlic, minced

- Salt and pepper to taste

- Fresh parsley for garnish

Directions:

1. Preheat oven to 375°F (190°C).

2. Place cod fillets in a baking dish.

3. In a small bowl, mix melted butter, lemon juice, lemon zest, and garlic. Pour over the cod fillets.

4. Season with salt and pepper.

5. Bake for 15-20 minutes, or until the cod flakes easily with a fork.

6. Garnish with fresh parsley and serve.

Nutrition (per serving):

- Calories: 250

- Protein: 25g

- Carbohydrates: 2g

- Fat: 16g

- Fiber: 1g

- Sodium: 250mg

Soft and Tender Chicken Pot Pie

Preparation Time: 20 minutes

Cooking Time: 45 minutes

Servings: 6

Ingredients:

- 2 cups cooked chicken, diced

- 1 cup frozen peas and carrots

- 1/2 cup celery, chopped

- 1/3 cup butter

- 1/3 cup all-purpose flour

- 1/2 teaspoon salt

- 1/4 teaspoon black pepper

- 1/4 teaspoon onion powder

- 1/4 teaspoon garlic powder

- 1 3/4 cups chicken broth

- 2/3 cup milk

- 1 package refrigerated pie crusts (2 crusts)

Directions:

1. Preheat oven to 425°F (220°C).

2. In a large saucepan, melt butter over medium heat. Add flour, salt, pepper, onion powder, and garlic powder. Stir until well blended.

3. Gradually stir in chicken broth and milk. Cook, stirring constantly, until the mixture thickens and boils.

4. Stir in chicken, peas, carrots, and celery. Remove from heat.

5. Fit one pie crust into the bottom of a 9-inch pie dish. Pour the chicken mixture into the crust.

6. Cover with the second crust, seal the edges, and cut slits in the top to allow steam to escape.

7. Bake for 30-35 minutes, or until the crust is golden brown. Let cool for 10 minutes before serving.

Nutrition (per serving):

- Calories: 450

- Protein: 20g

- Carbohydrates: 40g

- Fat: 22g

- Fiber: 3g

- Sodium: 600mg

Easy-to-Chew Quiche Lorraine

Preparation Time: 15 minutes

Cooking Time: 45 minutes

Servings: 6

Ingredients:

- 1 refrigerated pie crust

- 6 slices bacon, cooked and crumbled

- 1 cup shredded Swiss cheese

- 1/4 cup grated Parmesan cheese

- 1/2 cup onion, finely chopped

- 4 large eggs

- 1 cup half-and-half

- 1/4 teaspoon salt

- 1/4 teaspoon black pepper

- 1/4 teaspoon ground nutmeg

Directions:

1. Preheat oven to 375°F (190°C).

2. Fit pie crust into a 9-inch pie dish and crimp the edges.

3. Sprinkle bacon, Swiss cheese, Parmesan cheese, and onion evenly over the bottom of the pie crust.

4. In a medium bowl, whisk together eggs, half-and-half, salt, pepper, and nutmeg. Pour over the bacon and cheese.

5. Bake for 40-45 minutes, or until the quiche is set and the top is golden brown. Let cool for 10 minutes before slicing and serving.

Nutrition (per serving):

- Calories: 350

- Protein: 15g

- Carbohydrates: 20g

- Fat: 25g

- Fiber: 1g

- Sodium: 700mg

Tender Beef and Vegetable Stir-Fry

Preparation Time: 15 minutes

Cooking Time: 15 minutes

Servings: 4

Ingredients:

- 1 lb beef sirloin, thinly sliced

- 2 tablespoons soy sauce

- 1 tablespoon cornstarch

- 1 tablespoon vegetable oil

- 1 cup broccoli florets

- 1 cup bell peppers, sliced

- 1 cup snap peas

- 1/2 cup carrots, thinly sliced

- 3 cloves garlic, minced

- 1 tablespoon fresh ginger, grated

- 1/4 cup beef broth

- 2 tablespoons oyster sauce

- 1 teaspoon sesame oil

- Cooked rice for serving

Directions:

1. In a bowl, combine beef, soy sauce, and cornstarch. Mix well and set aside for 10 minutes.

2. Heat vegetable oil in a large skillet or wok over medium-high heat. Add beef and stir-fry until browned, then remove and set aside.

3. Add broccoli, bell peppers, snap peas, and carrots to the skillet. Stir-fry for 3-4 minutes.

4. Add garlic and ginger, and cook for another minute.

5. Return beef to the skillet. Add beef broth, oyster sauce, and sesame oil. Stir-fry for another 2-3 minutes, until everything is well coated and heated through.

6. Serve over cooked rice.

Nutrition (per serving):

- Calories: 300

- Protein: 25g

- Carbohydrates: 15g

- Fat: 15g

- Fiber: 4g

- Sodium: 800mg

Soft and Creamy Cauliflower Mac and Cheese

Preparation Time:10 minutes

Cooking Time: 20 minutes

Servings:4

Ingredients:

- 1 large head cauliflower, cut into florets

- 1/4 cup butter

- 1/4 cup all-purpose flour

- 2 cups milk

- 2 cups shredded cheddar cheese

- 1/2 teaspoon salt

- 1/4 teaspoon black pepper

- 1/4 teaspoon garlic powder (optional)

Directions:

1. Steam or boil cauliflower florets until tender, about 10 minutes. Drain and set aside.

2. In a saucepan, melt butter over medium heat. Stir in flour and cook for 1-2 minutes until smooth and bubbly.

3. Gradually add milk, stirring constantly until the mixture thickens.

4. Add cheddar cheese, salt, pepper, and garlic powder. Stir until cheese is melted and the sauce is smooth.

5. Combine the cheese sauce with the cooked cauliflower. Mix well and serve warm.

Nutrition (per serving):

- Calories: 300

- Protein: 14g

- Carbohydrates: 12g

- Fat: 22g

- Fiber: 3g

- Sodium: 500mg

Preparation Time: 10 minutes

Cooking Time: 10 minutes

Servings: 4

Ingredients:

- 1 lb large shrimp, peeled and deveined

- 3 tablespoons butter

- 3 tablespoons olive oil

- 4 cloves garlic, minced

- 1/4 cup dry white wine or chicken broth

- 1/4 cup lemon juice

- 1/4 teaspoon red pepper flakes (optional)

- Salt and pepper to taste

- 1/4 cup chopped fresh parsley

- Cooked pasta or crusty bread for serving

Directions:

1. Heat butter and olive oil in a large skillet over medium-high heat.

2. Add garlic and cook until fragrant, about 1 minute.

3. Add shrimp and cook until pink and opaque, about 2-3 minutes per side.

4. Remove shrimp from the skillet and set aside.

5. Add wine (or broth) and lemon juice to the skillet. Simmer for 2 minutes, scraping up any browned bits from the bottom.

6. Return shrimp to the skillet and toss to coat in the sauce. Season with red pepper flakes (if using), salt, and pepper.

7. Sprinkle with fresh parsley and serve over pasta or with crusty bread.

Nutrition (per serving):

- Calories: 300

- Protein: 25g

- Carbohydrates: 5g

- Fat: 18g

- Fiber: 0g

- Sodium: 600mg

Soft and Tender Pork Tenderloin with Apples

Preparation Time:15 minutes

Cooking Time: 30 minutes

Servings:4

Ingredients:

- 1 1/2 lb pork tenderloin

- 2 tablespoons olive oil

- 2 apples, peeled, cored, and sliced

- 1 onion, thinly sliced

- 2 tablespoons brown sugar

- 1/2 cup apple cider

- 1 teaspoon dried thyme

- Salt and pepper to taste

Directions:

1. Preheat oven to 375°F (190°C).

2. Season pork tenderloin with salt and pepper.

3. In a large oven-safe skillet, heat olive oil over medium-high heat. Sear the pork on all sides until browned, about 5 minutes.

4. Remove pork from the skillet and set aside.

5. Add apples and onion to the skillet. Sauté until softened, about 5 minutes.

6. Stir in brown sugar, apple cider, and thyme. Bring to a simmer.

7. Return pork to the skillet and spoon some of the apple mixture over the top.

8. Transfer the skillet to the oven and bake for 20-25 minutes, or until the internal temperature of the pork reaches 145°F (63°C).

9. Let the pork rest for 5 minutes before slicing. Serve with the apple mixture.

Nutrition (per serving):

- Calories: 350

- Protein: 30g

- Carbohydrates: 20g

- Fat: 15g

- Fiber: 3g

- Sodium: 250mg

Preparation Time:10 minutes

Cooking Time:20 minutes

Servings: 4

Ingredients:

- 8 oz fettuccine pasta

- 2 tablespoons butter

- 2 cloves garlic, minced

- 1 cup heavy cream

- 1 cup grated Parmesan cheese

- 1/2 teaspoon salt

- 1/4 teaspoon black pepper

- 2 cups cooked chicken, shredded or diced

- Fresh parsley for garnish

Directions:

1. Cook fettuccine according to package directions. Drain and set aside.

2. In a large skillet, melt butter over medium heat. Add garlic and cook until fragrant, about 1 minute.

3. Stir in heavy cream and bring to a simmer.

4. Gradually add Parmesan cheese, stirring until the sauce is smooth and thickened.

5. Season with salt and pepper.

6. Add cooked chicken and pasta to the skillet. Toss to coat in the Alfredo sauce.

7. Garnish with fresh parsley and serve warm.

Nutrition (per serving):

- Calories: 600

- Protein: 30g

- Carbohydrates: 45g

- Fat: 35g

- Fiber: 2g

- Sodium: 600mg

Moist and Tender Meatloaf Muffins

Preparation Time:15 minutes

Cooking Time:25 minutes

Servings: 6

Ingredients:

- 1 lb ground beef

- 1/2 cup breadcrumbs

- 1/2 cup milk

- 1 egg

- 1 small onion, finely chopped

- 2 cloves garlic, minced

- 1/4 cup ketchup

- 1 tablespoon Worcestershire sauce

- 1 teaspoon salt

- 1/2 teaspoon black pepper

- 1/4 cup grated Parmesan cheese (optional)

 Directions:

1. Preheat oven to 375°F (190°C). Grease a 12-cup muffin tin.

2. In a large bowl, combine all ingredients. Mix until well blended.

3. Divide the meat mixture evenly among the muffin cups.

4. Bake for 20-25 minutes, or until the internal temperature reaches 160°F (71°C).

5. Let rest for 5 minutes before serving.

Nutrition (per serving):

- Calories: 250

- Protein: 20g

- Carbohydrates: 10g

- Fat: 15g

- Fiber: 1g

- Sodium: 500mg

<h1 style="text-align:center">Chapter 4:</h1>

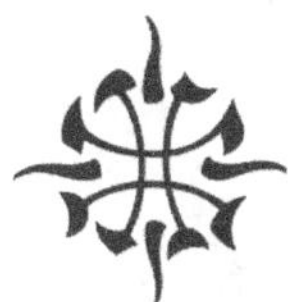

Thick and Hearty Chicken Noodle Soup

Preparation Time: 20 minutes

Cooking Time: 1 hour

Servings:6

Ingredients:

- 1 tablespoon olive oil

- 1 onion, chopped

- 3 cloves garlic, minced

- 3 carrots, peeled and sliced

- 3 celery stalks, sliced

- 8 cups chicken broth

- 2 cups cooked chicken, shredded

- 2 cups egg noodles

- 1 teaspoon dried thyme

- 1 teaspoon dried parsley

- 1 bay leaf

- Salt and pepper to taste

- 1/4 cup cornstarch mixed with 1/4 cup cold water (for thickening)

Directions:

1. Heat olive oil in a large pot over medium heat. Add onion, garlic, carrots, and celery. Sauté until vegetables are softened, about 5-7 minutes.

2. Add chicken broth, cooked chicken, thyme, parsley, bay leaf, salt, and pepper. Bring to a boil.

3. Reduce heat and simmer for 30 minutes.

4. Add egg noodles and cook for another 10 minutes, or until noodles are tender.

5. Stir in the cornstarch mixture and cook until the soup thickens, about 2-3 minutes.

6. Remove the bay leaf and serve hot.

Nutrition (per serving):

- Calories: 250

- Protein: 20g

- Carbohydrates: 25g

- Fat: 8g

- Fiber: 3g

- Sodium: 750mg

Creamy Thickened Tomato Soup

Preparation Time: 10 minutes

Cooking Time:30 minutes

Servings: 4

Ingredients:

- 2 tablespoons butter

- 1 onion, chopped

- 3 cloves garlic, minced

- 1 (28 oz) can crushed tomatoes

- 2 cups chicken broth

- 1 cup heavy cream

- 1 teaspoon sugar

- 1/2 teaspoon dried basil

- Salt and pepper to taste

- 2 tablespoons cornstarch mixed with 2 tablespoons cold water (for thickening)

Directions:

1. In a large pot, melt butter over medium heat. Add onion and garlic and sauté until softened, about 5 minutes.

2. Add crushed tomatoes, chicken broth, sugar, basil, salt, and pepper. Bring to a boil.

3. Reduce heat and simmer for 20 minutes.

4. Stir in the heavy cream and cornstarch mixture. Simmer until the soup thickens, about 5 minutes.

5. Use an immersion blender to blend the soup until smooth, if desired.

6. Serve hot.

Nutrition (per serving):

- Calories: 300

- Protein: 5g

- Carbohydrates: 20g

- Fat: 22g

- Fiber: 3g

- Sodium: 700mg

Rich and Thickened Beef Stew

Preparation Time: 20 minutes

Cooking Time:2 hours

Servings: 6

 Ingredients:

- 2 lb beef stew meat, cut into 1-inch cubes

- 2 tablespoons olive oil

- 1 onion, chopped

- 3 cloves garlic, minced

- 4 carrots, peeled and cut into chunks

- 4 potatoes, peeled and cut into chunks

- 2 cups beef broth

- 1 cup red wine (optional)

- 2 tablespoons tomato paste

- 1 teaspoon dried thyme

- 1 teaspoon dried rosemary

- 1 bay leaf

- Salt and pepper to taste

- 1/4 cup all-purpose flour mixed with 1/4 cup cold water (for thickening)

Directions:

1. In a large pot, heat olive oil over medium-high heat. Brown the beef on all sides, then remove and set aside.

2. Add onion and garlic to the pot and sauté until softened.

3. Stir in beef broth, red wine (if using), tomato paste, thyme, rosemary, bay leaf, salt, and pepper. Bring to a boil.

4. Return beef to the pot and add carrots and potatoes.

5. Reduce heat, cover, and simmer for 1.5 to 2 hours, or until the beef is tender.

6. Stir in the flour mixture and cook until the stew thickens, about 5 minutes.

7. Remove the bay leaf and serve hot.

 Nutrition (per serving):

- Calories: 450

- Protein: 35g

- Carbohydrates: 30g

- Fat: 20g

- Fiber: 5g

- Sodium: 700mg

Thickened Cream of Broccoli Soup

Preparation Time: 10 minutes

Cooking Time: 30 minutes

Servings: 4

Ingredients:

- 2 tablespoons butter

- 1 onion, chopped

- 3 cloves garlic, minced

- 4 cups broccoli florets

- 4 cups chicken or vegetable broth

- 1 cup heavy cream

- Salt and pepper to taste

- 2 tablespoons cornstarch mixed with 2 tablespoons cold water (for thickening)

- 1/2 cup shredded cheddar cheese (optional)

Directions:

1. In a large pot, melt butter over medium heat. Add onion and garlic and sauté until softened, about 5 minutes.

2. Add broccoli and broth. Bring to a boil, then reduce heat and simmer until the broccoli is tender, about 10-15 minutes.

3. Use an immersion blender to blend the soup until smooth.

4. Stir in the heavy cream and cornstarch mixture. Simmer until the soup thickens, about 5 minutes.

5. Season with salt and pepper. Stir in cheddar cheese, if using, until melted.

6. Serve hot.

Nutrition (per serving):

- Calories: 300

- Protein: 10g

- Carbohydrates: 20g

- Fat: 22g

- Fiber: 4g

- Sodium: 600mg

Flavorful Thickened Mushroom Gravy

Preparation Time: 10 minutes

Cooking Time: 20 minutes

Servings: 4

Ingredients:

- 2 tablespoons butter

- 1 onion, finely chopped

- 2 cloves garlic, minced

- 8 oz mushrooms, sliced

- 2 tablespoons all-purpose flour

- 2 cups beef or vegetable broth

- 1 teaspoon Worcestershire sauce

- Salt and pepper to taste

- 2 tablespoons cornstarch mixed with 2 tablespoons cold water (for thickening)

Directions:

1. In a large skillet, melt butter over medium heat. Add onion and garlic and sauté until softened.

2. Add mushrooms and cook until they release their juices and become tender, about 5-7 minutes.

3. Stir in flour and cook for 1-2 minutes until the flour is well incorporated.

4. Gradually add broth, stirring constantly. Bring to a simmer.

5. Add Worcestershire sauce, salt, and pepper. Stir well.

6. Stir in the cornstarch mixture and cook until the gravy thickens, about 2-3 minutes.

7. Serve hot over meats or mashed potatoes.

Nutrition (per serving):

- Calories: 100

- Protein: 3g

- Carbohydrates: 10g

- Fat: 5g

- Fiber: 1g

- Sodium: 500mg

Creamy Thickened Clam Chowder

Preparation Time: 15 minutes

Cooking Time: 30 minutes

Servings: 4

 Ingredients:

- 4 slices bacon, chopped

- 1 onion, finely chopped

- 2 cloves garlic, minced

- 3 potatoes, peeled and diced

- 2 cups clam juice

- 1 cup water

- 1 teaspoon dried thyme

- 1 bay leaf

- 2 (6.5 oz) cans chopped clams, with juice

- 1 cup heavy cream

- Salt and pepper to taste

- 2 tablespoons cornstarch mixed with 2 tablespoons cold water (for thickening)

Directions:

1. In a large pot, cook bacon over medium heat until crispy. Remove bacon and set aside, leaving the drippings in the pot.

2. Add onion and garlic to the pot and sauté until softened.

3. Add potatoes, clam juice, water, thyme, and bay leaf. Bring to a boil, then reduce heat and simmer until potatoes are tender, about 15 minutes.

4. Stir in clams with their juice and heavy cream. Heat through.

5. Stir in the cornstarch mixture and cook until the chowder thickens, about 5 minutes.

6. Season with salt and pepper. Remove bay leaf before serving. Top with reserved bacon.

Nutrition (per serving):

- Calories: 400

- Protein: 20g

- Carbohydrates: 35g

- Fat: 20g

- Fiber: 3g

- Sodium: 900mg

Thickened Potato and Bacon Soup

Preparation Time: 15 minutes

Cooking Time:30 minutes

Servings: 4

Ingredients:

- 6 slices bacon, chopped

- 1 onion, finely chopped

- 2 cloves garlic, minced

- 4 large potatoes, peeled and diced

- 4 cups chicken broth

- 1 cup milk

- 1 cup shredded cheddar cheese (optional)

- Salt and pepper to taste

- 2 tablespoons cornstarch mixed with 2 tablespoons cold water (for thickening)

- Chopped chives for garnish (optional)

Directions:

1. In a large pot, cook bacon over medium heat until crispy. Remove bacon and set aside, leaving the drippings in the pot.

2. Add onion and garlic to the pot and sauté until softened.

3. Add potatoes and chicken broth. Bring to a boil, then reduce heat and simmer until potatoes are tender, about 15 minutes.

4. Use a potato masher to slightly mash the potatoes, leaving some chunks.

5. Stir in milk and cheddar cheese (if using). Heat through.

6. Stir in the cornstarch mixture and cook until the soup thickens, about 5 minutes.

7. Season with salt and pepper. Garnish with cooked bacon and chives before serving.

Nutrition (per serving):

- Calories: 450

- Protein: 20g

- Carbohydrates: 45g

- Fat: 20g

- Fiber: 4g

- Sodium: 800mg

Chunky Thickened Vegetable Soup

Preparation Time: 15 minutes

Cooking Time: 40 minutes

Servings: 6

Ingredients:

- 2 tablespoons olive oil

- 1 onion, chopped

- 3 cloves garlic, minced

- 3 carrots, peeled and chopped

- 3 celery stalks, chopped

- 2 potatoes, peeled and diced

- 1 zucchini, chopped

- 1 cup green beans, chopped

- 1 (28 oz) can diced tomatoes

- 6 cups vegetable broth

- 1 teaspoon dried basil

- 1 teaspoon dried oregano

- Salt and pepper to taste

- 2 tablespoons cornstarch mixed with 2 tablespoons cold water (for thickening)

Directions:

1. Heat olive oil in a large pot over medium heat. Add onion and garlic and sauté until softened.

2. Add carrots, celery, potatoes, zucchini, and green beans. Cook for 5-7 minutes.

3. Stir in diced tomatoes, vegetable broth, basil, oregano, salt, and pepper. Bring to a boil.

4. Reduce heat and simmer for 25-30 minutes, or until vegetables are tender.

5. Stir in the cornstarch mixture and cook until the soup thickens, about 5 minutes.

6. Serve hot.

Nutrition (per serving):

- Calories: 200

- Protein: 5g

- Carbohydrates: 30g

- Fat: 7g

- Fiber: 7g

- Sodium: 600mg

Preparation Time: 15 minutes

Cooking Time:40 minutes

Servings: 6

 Ingredients:

- 2 tablespoons butter

- 1 onion, chopped

- 3 cloves garlic, minced

- 2 carrots, peeled and sliced

- 2 celery stalks, sliced

- 1 cup long-grain rice

- 8 cups chicken broth

- 2 cups cooked chicken, shredded

- 1 cup heavy cream

- 1 teaspoon dried thyme

- Salt and pepper to taste

- 2 tablespoons cornstarch mixed with 2 tablespoons cold water (for thickening)

Directions:

1. In a large pot, melt butter over medium heat. Add onion, garlic, carrots, and celery. Sauté until vegetables are softened, about 5-7 minutes.

2. Add rice and chicken broth. Bring to a boil, then reduce heat and simmer until rice is tender, about 20 minutes.

3. Stir in shredded chicken, heavy cream, thyme, salt, and pepper. Heat through.

4. Stir in the cornstarch mixture and cook until the soup thickens, about 5 minutes.

5. Serve hot.

Nutrition (per serving):

- Calories: 350

- Protein: 20g

- Carbohydrates: 40g

- Fat: 15g

- Fiber: 3g

- Sodium: 750mg

<hr>

Tangy Thickened Barbecue Sauce

Preparation Time:5 minutes

Cooking Time: 15 minutes

Servings: 2 cups

 Ingredients:

- 1 cup ketchup

- 1/2 cup apple cider vinegar

- 1/4 cup brown sugar

- 2 tablespoons Worcestershire sauce

- 2 tablespoons mustard

- 2 teaspoons smoked paprika

- 1 teaspoon garlic powder

- 1 teaspoon onion powder

- 1/2 teaspoon salt

- 1/2 teaspoon black pepper

- 1 tablespoon cornstarch mixed with 1 tablespoon cold water (for thickening)

Directions:

1. In a medium saucepan, combine all ingredients except the cornstarch mixture. Bring to a boil over medium heat.

2. Reduce heat and simmer for 10 minutes, stirring occasionally.

3. Stir in the cornstarch mixture and cook until the sauce thickens, about 2-3 minutes.

4. Let cool slightly before using. Store in the refrigerator.

Nutrition (per serving - 2 tablespoons):

- Calories: 50

- Protein: 0g

- Carbohydrates: 12g

- Fat: 0g

- Fiber: 0g

- Sodium: 200mg

Thickened Cream of Asparagus Soup

Preparation Time: 10 minutes

Cooking Time: 30 minutes

Servings: 4

Ingredients:

- 2 tablespoons butter

- 1 onion, chopped

- 3 cloves garlic, minced

- 1 lb asparagus, trimmed and chopped

- 4 cups chicken or vegetable broth

- 1 cup heavy cream

- Salt and pepper to taste

- 2 tablespoons cornstarch mixed with 2 tablespoons cold water (for thickening)

Directions:

1. In a large pot, melt butter over medium heat. Add onion and garlic and sauté until softened.

2. Add asparagus and broth. Bring to a boil, then reduce heat and simmer until asparagus is tender, about 15 minutes.

3. Use an immersion blender to blend the soup until smooth.

4. Stir in heavy cream, salt, and pepper. Heat through.

5. Stir in the cornstarch mixture and cook until the soup thickens, about 5 minutes.

6. Serve hot.

Nutrition (per serving):

- Calories: 300

- Protein: 5g

- Carbohydrates: 15g

- Fat: 25g

- Fiber: 4g

- Sodium: 600mg

Rich and Thickened Onion Gravy

Preparation Time: 10 minutes

Cooking Time: 30 minutes

Servings: 4

Ingredients:

- 2 tablespoons butter

- 2 large onions, thinly sliced

- 3 cloves garlic, minced

- 1 tablespoon all-purpose flour

- 2 cups beef broth

- 1 teaspoon Worcestershire sauce

- 1/2 teaspoon dried thyme

- Salt and pepper to taste

- 2 tablespoons cornstarch mixed with 2 tablespoons cold water (for thickening)

Directions:

1. In a large skillet, melt butter over medium heat. Add onions and cook, stirring frequently, until they are caramelized and golden brown, about 15-20 minutes.

2. Add garlic and cook for another minute.

3. Stir in flour and cook for 1-2 minutes until well incorporated.

4. Gradually add beef broth, stirring constantly. Bring to a simmer.

5. Add Worcestershire sauce, thyme, salt, and pepper. Stir well.

6. Stir in the cornstarch mixture and cook until the gravy thickens, about 5 minutes.

7. Serve hot over mashed potatoes or meat.

Nutrition (per serving):

- Calories: 100

- Protein: 2g

- Carbohydrates: 10g

- Fat: 5g

- Fiber: 1g

- Sodium: 500mg

Thickened Creamy Corn Chowder

Preparation Time: 15 minutes

Cooking Time: 30 minutes

Servings: 6

Ingredients:

- 4 slices bacon, chopped

- 1 onion, chopped

- 3 cloves garlic, minced

- 2 cups corn kernels (fresh or frozen)

- 2 potatoes, peeled and diced

- 4 cups chicken broth

- 1 cup heavy cream

- 1 teaspoon dried thyme

- Salt and pepper to taste

- 2 tablespoons cornstarch mixed with 2 tablespoons cold water (for thickening)

- 1/4 cup chopped fresh parsley (optional)

Directions:

1. In a large pot, cook bacon over medium heat until crispy. Remove bacon and set aside, leaving the drippings in the pot.

2. Add onion and garlic to the pot and sauté until softened, about 5 minutes.

3. Add corn, potatoes, and chicken broth. Bring to a boil, then reduce heat and simmer until potatoes are tender, about 15 minutes.

4. Stir in heavy cream, thyme, salt, and pepper. Heat through.

5. Stir in the cornstarch mixture and cook until the chowder thickens, about 5 minutes.

6. Garnish with cooked bacon and fresh parsley before serving.

Nutrition (per serving):

- Calories: 350

- Protein: 10g

- Carbohydrates: 40g

- Fat: 20g

- Fiber: 4g

- Sodium: 750mg

Flavorful Thickened Tomato Basil Sauce

Preparation Time:10 minutes

Cooking Time: 30 minutes

Servings:4

Ingredients:

- 2 tablespoons olive oil

- 1 onion, finely chopped

- 4 cloves garlic, minced

- 1 (28 oz) can crushed tomatoes

- 1 teaspoon sugar

- 1 teaspoon dried oregano

- 1/2 teaspoon salt

- 1/2 teaspoon black pepper

- 1/4 cup fresh basil leaves, chopped

- 2 tablespoons cornstarch mixed with 2 tablespoons cold water (for thickening)

Directions:

1. Heat olive oil in a large saucepan over medium heat. Add onion and garlic and sauté until softened, about 5 minutes.

2. Stir in crushed tomatoes, sugar, oregano, salt, and pepper. Bring to a boil, then reduce heat and simmer for 20 minutes.

3. Stir in fresh basil.

4. Stir in the cornstarch mixture and cook until the sauce thickens, about 5 minutes.

5. Serve hot over pasta or use as a base for other dishes.

Nutrition (per serving):

- Calories: 150

- Protein: 2g

- Carbohydrates: 15g

- Fat: 9g

- Fiber: 3g

- Sodium: 400mg

Thickened Cream of Cauliflower Soup

Preparation Time: 10 minutes

Cooking Time: 30 minutes

Servings: 4

Ingredients:

- 2 tablespoons butter

- 1 onion, chopped

- 3 cloves garlic, minced

- 1 large head cauliflower, chopped

- 4 cups chicken or vegetable broth

- 1 cup heavy cream

- Salt and pepper to taste

- 2 tablespoons cornstarch mixed with 2 tablespoons cold water (for thickening)

- 1/4 cup grated Parmesan cheese (optional)

- Chopped chives for garnish (optional)

Directions:

1. In a large pot, melt butter over medium heat. Add onion and garlic and sauté until softened, about 5 minutes.

2. Add cauliflower and broth. Bring to a boil, then reduce heat and simmer until cauliflower is tender, about 15 minutes.

3. Use an immersion blender to blend the soup until smooth.

4. Stir in heavy cream, salt, and pepper. Heat through.

5. Stir in the cornstarch mixture and cook until the soup thickens, about 5 minutes.

6. Stir in Parmesan cheese, if using. Garnish with chopped chives before serving.

Nutrition (per serving):

- Calories: 300

- Protein: 5g

- Carbohydrates: 15g

- Fat: 25g

- Fiber: 4g

- Sodium: 600mg

Tangy Thickened Honey Mustard Sauce

Preparation Time: 5 minutes

Cooking Time: 5 minutes

Servings: 1 cup

Ingredients:

- 1/2 cup Dijon mustard

- 1/4 cup honey

- 1/4 cup mayonnaise

- 1 tablespoon apple cider vinegar

- 1 teaspoon garlic powder

- 1 teaspoon onion powder

- Salt and pepper to taste

- 1 tablespoon cornstarch mixed with 1 tablespoon cold water (for thickening)

Directions:

1. In a small saucepan, combine Dijon mustard, honey, mayonnaise, apple cider vinegar, garlic powder, onion powder, salt, and pepper. Whisk until smooth.

2. Heat over medium heat until the mixture begins to simmer.

3. Stir in the cornstarch mixture and cook until the sauce thickens, about 2-3 minutes.

4. Remove from heat and let cool slightly before serving. Store in the refrigerator.

Nutrition (per serving - 2 tablespoons):

- Calories: 100

- Protein: 1g

- Carbohydrates: 12g

- Fat: 6g

- Fiber: 0g

- Sodium: 300mg

Preparation Time: 20 minutes

Cooking Time:1 hour

Servings: 6

Ingredients:

- 2 tablespoons olive oil

- 1 onion, chopped

- 3 cloves garlic, minced

- 1 lb ground beef

- 1 red bell pepper, chopped

- 1 green bell pepper, chopped

- 1 (28 oz) can crushed tomatoes

- 2 cups beef broth

- 1 (15 oz) can kidney beans, drained and rinsed

- 1 (15 oz) can black beans, drained and rinsed

- 2 tablespoons chili powder

- 1 teaspoon ground cumin

- 1 teaspoon smoked paprika

- 1/2 teaspoon dried oregano

- Salt and pepper to taste

- 2 tablespoons cornstarch mixed with 2 tablespoons cold water (for thickening)

- Shredded cheddar cheese and chopped green onions for garnish (optional)

Directions:

1. In a large pot, heat olive oil over medium heat. Add onion and garlic and sauté until softened, about 5 minutes.

2. Add ground beef and cook until browned, breaking it apart with a spoon.

3. Add red and green bell peppers and cook for another 5 minutes.

4. Stir in crushed tomatoes, beef broth, kidney beans, black beans, chili powder, cumin, smoked paprika, oregano, salt, and pepper. Bring to a boil.

5. Reduce heat and simmer for 45 minutes, stirring occasionally.

6. Stir in the cornstarch mixture and cook until the chili thickens, about 5 minutes.

7. Serve hot, garnished with shredded cheddar cheese and chopped green onions if desired.

Nutrition (per serving):

- Calories: 350

- Protein: 25g

- Carbohydrates: 30g

- Fat: 15g

- Fiber: 8g

- Sodium: 800mg

Thickened Creamy Spinach and Artichoke Soup

Preparation Time:15 minutes

Cooking Time: 30 minutes

Servings: 4

Ingredients:

- 2 tablespoons butter

- 1 onion, chopped

- 3 cloves garlic, minced

- 1 (14 oz) can artichoke hearts, drained and chopped

- 4 cups fresh spinach, chopped

- 4 cups chicken or vegetable broth

- 1 cup heavy cream

- Salt and pepper to taste

- 2 tablespoons cornstarch mixed with 2 tablespoons cold water (for thickening)

- 1/2 cup grated Parmesan cheese

Directions:

1. In a large pot, melt butter over medium heat. Add onion and garlic and sauté until softened, about 5 minutes.

2. Add chopped artichoke hearts and spinach. Cook until the spinach wilts, about 3-5 minutes.

3. Stir in broth and bring to a boil. Reduce heat and simmer for 15 minutes.

4. Stir in heavy cream, salt, and pepper. Heat through.

5. Stir in the cornstarch mixture and cook until the soup thickens, about 5 minutes.

6. Stir in grated Parmesan cheese until melted and well combined.

7. Serve hot.

Nutrition (per serving):

- Calories: 300

- Protein: 10g

- Carbohydrates: 15g

- Fat: 25g

- Fiber: 4g

- Sodium: 700mg

Rich and Thickened Mushroom Sauce

Preparation Time:10 minutes

Cooking Time: 20 minutes

Servings: 4

Ingredients:

- 2 tablespoons butter

- 1 onion, finely chopped

- 3 cloves garlic, minced

- 10 oz mushrooms, sliced

- 1 cup beef or vegetable broth

- 1 cup heavy cream

- 1 teaspoon dried thyme

- Salt and pepper to taste

- 2 tablespoons cornstarch mixed with 2 tablespoons cold water (for thickening)

Directions:

1. In a large skillet, melt butter over medium heat. Add onion and garlic and sauté until softened, about 5 minutes.

2. Add mushrooms and cook until they release their juices and become tender, about 5-7 minutes.

3. Stir in broth and bring to a simmer.

4. Stir in heavy cream, thyme, salt, and pepper. Simmer for 5 minutes.

5. Stir in the cornstarch mixture and cook until the sauce thickens, about 2-3 minutes.

6. Serve hot over meats or pasta.

Nutrition (per serving):

- Calories: 250

- Protein: 4g

- Carbohydrates: 10g

- Fat: 22g

- Fiber: 1g

- Sodium: 400mg

Thickened Creamy Broccoli and Cheddar Soup

Preparation Time: 15 minutes

Cooking Time: 30 minutes

Servings:4

Ingredients:

- 2 tablespoons butter

- 1 onion, chopped

- 3 cloves garlic, minced

- 4 cups broccoli florets

- 4 cups chicken or vegetable broth

- 1 cup heavy cream

- 1 cup shredded cheddar cheese

- Salt and pepper to taste

- 2 tablespoons cornstarch mixed with 2 tablespoons cold water (for thickening)

Directions:

1. In a large pot, melt butter over medium heat. Add onion and garlic and sauté until softened, about 5 minutes.

2. Add broccoli and broth. Bring to a boil, then reduce heat and simmer until broccoli is tender, about 15 minutes.

3. Use an immersion blender to blend the soup until smooth.

4. Stir in heavy cream, shredded cheddar cheese, salt, and pepper. Heat through until cheese is melted.

5. Stir in the cornstarch mixture and cook until the soup thickens, about 5 minutes.

6. Serve hot.

Nutrition (per serving):

- Calories: 400

- Protein: 15g

- Carbohydrates: 20g

- Fat: 30g

- Fiber: 4g

- Sodium: 700mg

Chapter 5:

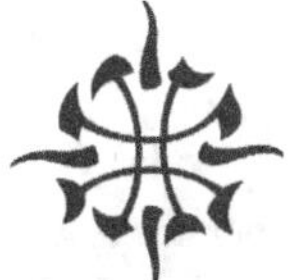

Easy-to-Swallow Banana Pudding

Preparation Time: 15 minutes

Chilling Time: 2 hours

Servings: 6

Ingredients:

- 2 cups whole milk

- 1/2 cup granulated sugar

- 1/4 cup cornstarch

- 1/4 teaspoon salt

- 3 egg yolks

- 1 teaspoon vanilla extract

- 3 ripe bananas, sliced

- Whipped cream for topping (optional)

Directions:

1. In a medium saucepan, whisk together milk, sugar, cornstarch, and salt. Cook over medium heat, stirring constantly, until the mixture thickens and begins to boil.

2. In a small bowl, whisk the egg yolks. Gradually whisk in a small amount of the hot milk mixture to temper the eggs, then pour the egg mixture back into the saucepan.

3. Cook for another 2 minutes, stirring constantly, until the pudding is thick and smooth.

4. Remove from heat and stir in vanilla extract.

5. Layer banana slices and pudding in serving dishes.

6. Chill in the refrigerator for at least 2 hours before serving. Top with whipped cream if desired.

Nutrition (per serving):

- Calories: 200

- Protein: 4g

- Carbohydrates: 38g

- Fat: 4g

- Fiber: 1g

- Sodium: 150mg

Moist and Soft Chocolate Mousse

Preparation Time: 20 minutes

Chilling Time: 2 hours

Servings: 6

Ingredients:

- 1 cup heavy cream

- 4 oz semi-sweet chocolate, chopped

- 2 tablespoons sugar

- 2 large eggs, separated

- 1 teaspoon vanilla extract

Directions:

1. In a medium saucepan, heat 1/2 cup of the heavy cream until just simmering. Remove from heat and add chopped chocolate, stirring until melted and smooth.

2. Whisk in sugar, egg yolks, and vanilla extract until well combined.

3. In a separate bowl, beat egg whites until stiff peaks form.

4. Fold egg whites into the chocolate mixture until fully incorporated.

5. In another bowl, whip the remaining 1/2 cup of heavy cream until soft peaks form, then fold into the chocolate mixture.

6. Spoon the mousse into serving dishes and refrigerate for at least 2 hours before serving.

Nutrition (per serving):

- Calories: 250

- Protein: 4g

- Carbohydrates: 20g

- Fat: 20g

- Fiber: 2g

- Sodium: 50mg

Soft and Creamy Rice Pudding

Preparation Time: 10 minutes

Cooking Time: 30 minutes

Servings: 4

Ingredients:

- 1/2 cup Arborio rice

- 4 cups whole milk

- 1/4 cup granulated sugar

- 1 teaspoon vanilla extract

- 1/4 teaspoon salt

- 1/2 teaspoon ground cinnamon (optional)

- Raisins for garnish (optional)

Directions:

1. In a medium saucepan, combine rice, milk, sugar, vanilla extract, and salt.

2. Cook over medium heat, stirring frequently, until the mixture thickens and rice is tender, about 30 minutes.

3. Remove from heat and let cool slightly.

4. Serve warm or chilled, sprinkled with ground cinnamon and garnished with raisins if desired.

Nutrition (per serving):

- Calories: 250

- Protein: 7g

- Carbohydrates: 45g

- Fat: 5g

- Fiber: 1g

- Sodium: 200mg

Tender Apple Cinnamon Bread Pudding

Preparation Time: 15 minutes

Cooking Time: 40 minutes

Servings: 6

Ingredients:

- 4 cups cubed bread (preferably day-old)

- 2 apples, peeled, cored, and chopped

- 2 cups whole milk

- 1/2 cup granulated sugar

- 2 large eggs

- 1 teaspoon vanilla extract

- 1 teaspoon ground cinnamon

- 1/4 teaspoon ground nutmeg

Directions:

1. Preheat oven to 350°F (175°C). Grease a baking dish.

2. In a large bowl, combine bread cubes and chopped apples.

3. In another bowl, whisk together milk, sugar, eggs, vanilla extract, cinnamon, and nutmeg.

4. Pour the milk mixture over the bread and apples, stirring to combine.

5. Transfer the mixture to the prepared baking dish and let sit for 10 minutes to soak.

6. Bake for 40 minutes, or until the pudding is set and the top is golden brown.

7. Serve warm.

Nutrition (per serving):

- Calories: 300

- Protein: 8g

- Carbohydrates: 50g

- Fat: 8g

- Fiber: 3g

- Sodium: 200mg

Smooth and Fluffy Strawberry Cheesecake

Preparation Time: 20 minutes

Chilling Time: 4 hours

Servings: 8

 Ingredients:

- 1 1/2 cups graham cracker crumbs

- 1/4 cup granulated sugar

- 1/2 cup butter, melted

- 16 oz cream cheese, softened

- 1 cup powdered sugar

- 1 teaspoon vanilla extract

- 1 cup heavy cream

- 1 cup fresh strawberries, pureed

Directions:

1. In a medium bowl, combine graham cracker crumbs, granulated sugar, and melted butter. Press the mixture into the bottom of a springform pan to form the crust.

2. In a large bowl, beat the cream cheese until smooth. Add powdered sugar and vanilla extract, and beat until well combined.

3. In a separate bowl, whip the heavy cream until stiff peaks form. Gently fold the whipped cream into the cream cheese mixture.

4. Fold in the pureed strawberries until fully incorporated.

5. Pour the mixture over the crust and smooth the top.

6. Refrigerate for at least 4 hours, or until set.

7. Serve chilled.

Nutrition (per serving):

- Calories: 450

- Protein: 5g

- Carbohydrates: 35g

- Fat: 35g

- Fiber: 1g

- Sodium: 300mg

Soft and Moist Carrot Cake Cupcakes

Preparation Time: 20 minutes

Cooking Time: 20 minutes

Servings:12 cupcakes

Ingredients:

- 1 1/2 cups all-purpose flour

- 1 teaspoon baking soda

- 1 teaspoon ground cinnamon

- 1/2 teaspoon ground nutmeg

- 1/2 teaspoon salt

- 2 large eggs

- 1 cup granulated sugar

- 1/2 cup vegetable oil

- 1/4 cup unsweetened applesauce

- 1 teaspoon vanilla extract

- 1 1/2 cups finely grated carrots

- 1/2 cup crushed pineapple, drained

- 1/2 cup chopped walnuts (optional)

- 8 oz cream cheese, softened

- 1/4 cup unsalted butter, softened

- 2 cups powdered sugar

- 1 teaspoon vanilla extract

Directions:

1. Preheat oven to 350°F (175°C). Line a muffin tin with cupcake liners.

2. In a bowl, whisk together flour, baking soda, cinnamon, nutmeg, and salt.

3. In another bowl, beat eggs and granulated sugar until thick and pale. Add oil, applesauce, and vanilla extract; mix until well combined.

4. Gradually add the dry ingredients to the wet ingredients, mixing until just combined. Fold in grated carrots, pineapple, and walnuts (if using).

5. Divide the batter evenly among the cupcake liners. Bake for 18-20 minutes, or until a toothpick inserted into the center comes out clean. Let cool completely.

6. For the frosting, beat cream cheese and butter until smooth. Gradually add powdered sugar and vanilla extract, beating until light and fluffy.

7. Frost the cooled cupcakes and serve.

Nutrition (per cupcake):

- Calories: 300

- Protein: 4g

- Carbohydrates: 40g

- Fat: 15g

- Fiber: 1g

- Sodium: 200mg

Creamy Vanilla Panna Cotta

Preparation Time: 10 minutes

Chilling Time: 4 hours

Servings: 4

Ingredients:

- 1 cup whole milk

- 1 cup heavy cream

- 1/3 cup granulated sugar

- 1 teaspoon vanilla extract

- 1 packet (1 tablespoon) unflavored gelatin

- 2 tablespoons cold water

- Fresh berries for garnish (optional)

Directions:

1. In a saucepan, combine milk, heavy cream, and sugar. Heat over medium heat until the sugar dissolves and the mixture is hot but not boiling.

2. Remove from heat and stir in vanilla extract.

3. In a small bowl, sprinkle gelatin over cold water and let sit for 5 minutes to bloom.

4. Stir the gelatin mixture into the hot milk mixture until completely dissolved.

5. Pour the mixture into serving dishes and refrigerate for at least 4 hours, or until set.

6. Serve chilled, topped with fresh berries if desired.

Nutrition (per serving):

- Calories: 250

- Protein: 5g

- Carbohydrates: 20g

- Fat: 20g

- Fiber: 0g

- Sodium: 50mg

Preparation Time: 15 minutes

Cooking Time: 40 minutes

Servings: 6

Ingredients:

- 4 cups fresh or frozen blueberries

- 1/2 cup granulated sugar

- 1 tablespoon lemon juice

- 1 teaspoon lemon zest

- 1 cup all-purpose flour

- 1/2 cup granulated sugar

- 1 teaspoon baking powder

- 1/2 teaspoon salt

- 1/2 cup milk

- 1/4 cup unsalted butter, melted

Directions:

1. Preheat oven to 375°F (190°C). Grease a baking dish.

2. In a bowl, combine blueberries, 1/2 cup sugar, lemon juice, and lemon zest. Pour into the prepared baking dish.

3. In another bowl, mix flour, 1/2 cup sugar, baking powder, and salt. Stir in milk and melted butter until just combined.

4. Drop spoonfuls of the batter over the blueberries, spreading gently to cover most of the fruit.

5. Bake for 35-40 minutes, or until the top is golden brown and the blueberries are bubbly.

6. Serve warm, optionally with a scoop of vanilla ice cream.

Nutrition (per serving):

- Calories: 300

- Protein: 3g

- Carbohydrates: 55g

- Fat: 10g

- Fiber: 4g

- Sodium: 200mg

Soft and Fluffy Lemon Bars

Preparation Time: 15 minutes

Cooking Time: 35 minutes

Servings: 12

Ingredients:

- 1 cup all-purpose flour

- 1/2 cup unsalted butter, softened

- 1/4 cup powdered sugar

- 1 cup granulated sugar

- 2 large eggs

- 2 tablespoons all-purpose flour

- 1/2 teaspoon baking powder

- 1/4 cup lemon juice

- 1 tablespoon lemon zest

- Powdered sugar for dusting

Directions:

1. Preheat oven to 350°F (175°C). Grease an 8x8-inch baking dish.

2. In a bowl, mix 1 cup flour, butter, and 1/4 cup powdered sugar until a dough forms. Press into the bottom of the prepared baking dish.

3. Bake for 15 minutes, or until lightly golden. Remove from oven and set aside.

4. In another bowl, whisk granulated sugar, eggs, 2 tablespoons flour, baking powder, lemon juice, and lemon zest until smooth.

5. Pour the lemon mixture over the baked crust.

6. Bake for an additional 20 minutes, or until the lemon layer is set.

7. Let cool completely, then dust with powdered sugar before cutting into bars.

Nutrition (per serving):

- Calories: 180

- Protein: 2g

- Carbohydrates: 28g

- Fat: 7g

- Fiber: 0g

- Sodium: 80mg

Moist and Tender Pumpkin Bread

Preparation Time: 15 minutes

Cooking Time: 60 minutes

Servings: 10

Ingredients:

- 1 3/4 cups all-purpose flour

- 1 teaspoon baking soda

- 1/2 teaspoon salt

- 1/2 teaspoon ground cinnamon

- 1/4 teaspoon ground nutmeg

- 1/4 teaspoon ground cloves

- 1/2 cup unsalted butter, softened

- 1 cup granulated sugar

- 2 large eggs

- 1 cup canned pumpkin puree

- 1/4 cup milk

- 1 teaspoon vanilla extract

Directions:

1. Preheat oven to 350°F (175°C). Grease a 9x5-inch loaf pan.

2. In a bowl, whisk together flour, baking soda, salt, cinnamon, nutmeg, and cloves.

3. In another bowl, beat butter and sugar until creamy. Add eggs one at a time, beating well after each addition.

4. Mix in pumpkin puree, milk, and vanilla extract.

5. Gradually add the dry ingredients to the wet ingredients, mixing until just combined.

6. Pour the batter into the prepared loaf pan and smooth the top.

7. Bake for 60 minutes, or until a toothpick inserted into the center comes out clean.

8. Let cool in the pan for 10 minutes, then transfer to a wire rack to cool completely.

Nutrition (per serving):

- Calories: 250

- Protein: 4g

- Carbohydrates: 38g

- Fat: 10g

- Fiber: 2g

- Sodium: 200mg

Creamy Chocolate Avocado Mousse

Preparation Time: 10 minutes

Chilling Time: 30 minutes

Servings: 4

Ingredients:

- 2 ripe avocados, peeled and pitted

- 1/2 cup unsweetened cocoa powder

- 1/2 cup maple syrup or honey

- 1/4 cup almond milk (or any milk of choice)

- 1 teaspoon vanilla extract

- Pinch of salt

- Fresh berries or mint leaves for garnish (optional)

Directions:

1. In a food processor, combine avocados, cocoa powder, maple syrup (or honey), almond milk, vanilla extract, and salt.

2. Blend until smooth and creamy.

3. Spoon the mousse into serving dishes and refrigerate for at least 30 minutes before serving.

4. Garnish with fresh berries or mint leaves if desired.

Nutrition (per serving):

- Calories: 250

- Protein: 3g

- Carbohydrates: 40g

- Fat: 14g

- Fiber: 7g

- Sodium: 50mg

Soft and Fluffy Coconut Macaroons

Preparation Time: 10 minutes

Cooking Time: 20 minutes

Servings: 12

Ingredients:

- 3 cups shredded coconut (sweetened or unsweetened)

- 1/2 cup sweetened condensed milk

- 1 teaspoon vanilla extract

- 2 large egg whites

- 1/4 teaspoon salt

Directions:

1. Preheat oven to 325°F (165°C). Line a baking sheet with parchment paper.

2. In a large bowl, mix shredded coconut, sweetened condensed milk, and vanilla extract until well combined.

3. In another bowl, beat egg whites and salt until stiff peaks form.

4. Gently fold the egg whites into the coconut mixture.

5. Drop tablespoonfuls of the mixture onto the prepared baking sheet.

6. Bake for 18-20 minutes, or until the macaroons are golden brown.

7. Let cool completely on a wire rack.

Nutrition (per macaroon):

- Calories: 140

- Protein: 2g

- Carbohydrates: 20g

- Fat: 7g

- Fiber: 3g

- Sodium: 50mg

Easy-to-Swallow Peach Melba

Preparation Time: 10 minutes

Chilling Time: 1 hour

Servings: 4

Ingredients:

- 4 ripe peaches, peeled and sliced

- 1/2 cup raspberry sauce (store-bought or homemade)

- 1 cup vanilla ice cream or Greek yogurt

- Fresh raspberries for garnish (optional)

- Mint leaves for garnish (optional)

Directions:

1. Arrange peach slices in serving dishes.

2. Drizzle raspberry sauce over the peaches.

3. Top with a scoop of vanilla ice cream or Greek yogurt.

4. Garnish with fresh raspberries and mint leaves if desired.

5. Chill in the refrigerator for 1 hour before serving.

Nutrition (per serving):

- Calories: 150

- Protein: 3g

- Carbohydrates: 30g

- Fat: 2g

- Fiber: 3g

- Sodium: 30mg

Tender Banana Bread with Cream Cheese Frosting

Preparation Time: 15 minutes

Cooking Time: 60 minutes

Servings: 10

Ingredients:

- 2 cups all-purpose flour

- 1 teaspoon baking soda

- 1/2 teaspoon salt

- 1/2 teaspoon ground cinnamon

- 1/2 cup unsalted butter, softened

- 1 cup granulated sugar

- 2 large eggs

- 1 teaspoon vanilla extract

- 4 ripe bananas, mashed

- 1/4 cup milk

- 8 oz cream cheese, softened

- 1/4 cup unsalted butter, softened

- 2 cups powdered sugar

- 1 teaspoon vanilla extract

Directions:

1. Preheat oven to 350°F (175°C). Grease a 9x5-inch loaf pan.

2. In a bowl, whisk together flour, baking soda, salt, and cinnamon.

3. In another bowl, beat butter and sugar until creamy. Add eggs one at a time, beating well after each addition.

4. Mix in vanilla extract, mashed bananas, and milk.

5. Gradually add the dry ingredients to the wet ingredients, mixing until just combined.

6. Pour the batter into the prepared loaf pan and smooth the top.

7. Bake for 60 minutes, or until a toothpick inserted into the center comes out clean.

8. Let cool in the pan for 10 minutes, then transfer to a wire rack to cool completely.

9. For the frosting, beat cream cheese and butter until smooth. Gradually add powdered sugar and vanilla extract, beating until light and fluffy.

10. Frost the cooled banana bread and serve.

Nutrition (per serving):

- Calories: 400

- Protein: 5g

- Carbohydrates: 60g

- Fat: 15g

- Fiber: 2g

- Sodium: 300mg

Soft and Creamy Tiramisu

Preparation Time: 30 minutes

Chilling Time: 4 hours

Servings: 8

Ingredients:

- 1 cup heavy cream

- 8 oz mascarpone cheese

- 1/2 cup granulated sugar

- 1 teaspoon vanilla extract

- 1 1/2 cups strong brewed coffee, cooled

- 2 tablespoons coffee liqueur (optional)

- 24 ladyfinger cookies

- Unsweetened cocoa powder for dusting

Directions:

1. In a bowl, beat heavy cream until stiff peaks form. Set aside.

2. In another bowl, beat mascarpone cheese, sugar, and vanilla extract until smooth and creamy.

3. Fold the whipped cream into the mascarpone mixture.

4. In a shallow dish, combine cooled coffee and coffee liqueur (if using).

5. Dip each ladyfinger briefly into the coffee mixture and arrange a single layer in the bottom of a 9x9-inch dish.

6. Spread half of the mascarpone mixture over the ladyfingers.

7. Repeat with another layer of dipped ladyfingers and the remaining mascarpone mixture.

8. Dust the top with unsweetened cocoa powder.

9. Refrigerate for at least 4 hours, or until set, before serving.

Nutrition (per serving):

- Calories: 350

- Protein: 5g

- Carbohydrates: 30g

- Fat: 25g

- Fiber: 1g

- Sodium: 100mg

Preparation Time: 20 minutes

Cooking Time: 20 minutes

Servings: 12 cupcakes

Ingredients:

- 1 1/4 cups all-purpose flour

- 1 cup granulated sugar

- 1 tablespoon unsweetened cocoa powder

- 1/2 teaspoon baking soda

- 1/2 teaspoon salt

- 1 large egg

- 3/4 cup vegetable oil

- 1/2 cup buttermilk

- 1 tablespoon red food coloring

- 1 teaspoon vanilla extract

- 1/2 teaspoon white vinegar

- 8 oz cream cheese, softened

- 1/4 cup unsalted butter, softened

- 2 cups powdered sugar

- 1 teaspoon vanilla extract

Directions:

1. Preheat oven to 350°F (175°C). Line a muffin tin with cupcake liners.

2. In a bowl, sift together flour, sugar, cocoa powder, baking soda, and salt.

3. In another bowl, whisk together egg, oil, buttermilk, red food coloring, vanilla extract, and vinegar.

4. Gradually add the dry ingredients to the wet ingredients, mixing until just combined.

5. Divide the batter evenly among the cupcake liners. Bake for 18-20 minutes, or until a toothpick inserted into the center comes out clean. Let cool completely.

6. For the frosting, beat cream cheese and butter until smooth. Gradually add powdered sugar and vanilla extract, beating until light and fluffy.

7. Frost the cooled cupcakes and serve.

Nutrition (per cupcake):

- Calories: 300

- Protein: 3g

- Carbohydrates: 40g

- Fat: 15g

- Fiber: 0g

- Sodium: 200mg

Smooth and Creamy Mango Pudding

Preparation Time: 15 minutes

Chilling Time: 2 hours

Servings: 4

Ingredients:

- 2 ripe mangoes, peeled and chopped

- 1/2 cup coconut milk

- 1/4 cup granulated sugar

- 1/2 cup water

- 1 tablespoon unflavored gelatin

- Fresh mint leaves for garnish (optional)

Directions:

1. In a blender, puree the mangoes until smooth. Set aside.

2. In a small saucepan, combine coconut milk, sugar, and water. Heat over medium heat until the sugar dissolves, then remove from heat.

3. Sprinkle gelatin over the mixture and stir until dissolved.

4. Stir in the mango puree until well combined.

5. Pour the mixture into serving dishes and refrigerate for at least 2 hours, or until set.

6. Garnish with fresh mint leaves if desired before serving.

Nutrition (per serving):

- Calories: 150

- Protein: 2g

- Carbohydrates: 30g

- Fat: 4g

- Fiber: 2g

- Sodium: 20mg

Soft and Fluffy Peanut Butter Cookies

Preparation Time:15 minutes

Cooking Time: 10 minutes

Servings: 24 cookies

Ingredients:

- 1 cup creamy peanut butter

- 1/2 cup granulated sugar

- 1/2 cup brown sugar, packed

- 1 large egg

- 1 teaspoon vanilla extract

- 1 teaspoon baking soda

- 1/4 teaspoon salt

Directions:

1. Preheat oven to 350°F (175°C). Line a baking sheet with parchment paper.

2. In a bowl, beat peanut butter, granulated sugar, and brown sugar until creamy.

3. Add egg and vanilla extract, and beat until well combined.

4. Stir in baking soda and salt until the dough is smooth.

5. Drop tablespoonfuls of dough onto the prepared baking sheet, flattening each slightly with a fork.

6. Bake for 10 minutes, or until the edges are lightly golden. Let cool on the baking sheet for a few minutes before transferring to a wire rack to cool completely.

Nutrition (per cookie):

  Calories: 100

- Protein: 2g

- Carbohydrates: 10g

- Fat: 6g

- Fiber: 1g

- Sodium: 90mg

Preparation Time: 20 minutes

Chilling Time: 2 hours

Servings:8

Ingredients:

- 1 chocolate cake mix, prepared and cooled

- 1 can (21 oz) cherry pie filling

- 2 cups whipped cream or whipped topping

- 1/4 cup grated chocolate (optional)

- Fresh cherries for garnish (optional)

Directions:

1. Cut the prepared chocolate cake into small cubes.

2. In a trifle bowl or large glass bowl, layer half of the cake cubes.

3. Spoon half of the cherry pie filling over the cake.

4. Spread half of the whipped cream over the cherry pie filling.

5. Repeat the layers with the remaining cake, cherry pie filling, and whipped cream.

6. Sprinkle grated chocolate on top and garnish with fresh cherries if desired.

7. Refrigerate for at least 2 hours before serving.

Nutrition (per serving):

- Calories: 300

- Protein: 3g

- Carbohydrates: 45g

- Fat: 15g

- Fiber: 2g

- Sodium: 250mg

Moist and Delicious Zucchini Bread

Preparation Time: 15 minutes

Cooking Time: 60 minutes

Servings: 10

Ingredients:

- 1 1/2 cups all-purpose flour

- 1/2 teaspoon baking powder

- 1/2 teaspoon baking soda

- 1/2 teaspoon salt

- 1/2 teaspoon ground cinnamon

- 1/4 teaspoon ground nutmeg

- 1/4 teaspoon ground cloves

- 1/2 cup vegetable oil

- 1/2 cup granulated sugar

- 1/2 cup brown sugar, packed

- 2 large eggs

- 1 teaspoon vanilla extract

- 1 1/2 cups grated zucchini

- 1/2 cup chopped walnuts (optional)

Directions:

1. Preheat oven to 350°F (175°C). Grease a 9x5-inch loaf pan.

2. In a bowl, whisk together flour, baking powder, baking soda, salt, cinnamon, nutmeg, and cloves.

3. In another bowl, beat oil, granulated sugar, and brown sugar until creamy. Add eggs one at a time, beating well after each addition.

4. Mix in vanilla extract and grated zucchini.

5. Gradually add the dry ingredients to the wet ingredients, mixing until just combined. Fold in walnuts if using.

6. Pour the batter into the prepared loaf pan and smooth the top.

7. Bake for 60 minutes, or until a toothpick inserted into the center comes out clean.

8. Let cool in the pan for 10 minutes, then transfer to a wire rack to cool completely.

Nutrition (per serving):

- Calories: 250

- Protein: 4g

- Carbohydrates: 35g

- Fat: 10g

- Fiber: 2g

- Sodium: 200mg

Chapter 6:

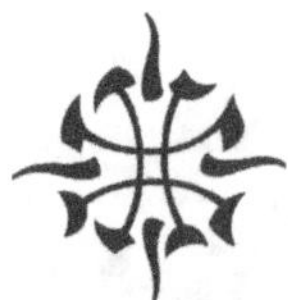

NUTRITIOUS AND REFRESHING BEVERAGES

Creamy and Nutritious Protein Shake

Preparation Time: 5 minutes

Servings: 1

Ingredients:

- 1 scoop protein powder (flavor of your choice)

- 1 cup unsweetened almond milk

- 1/2 banana

- 1 tablespoon peanut butter or almond butter

- 1/4 cup Greek yogurt

- 1 tablespoon honey or maple syrup

- Ice cubes (optional)

Directions:

1. Combine all ingredients in a blender.

2. Blend until smooth and creamy.

3. If desired, add ice cubes and blend again until desired consistency is reached.

4. Pour into a glass and enjoy immediately.

Nutrition (per serving):

- Calories: 300

- Protein: 25g

- Carbohydrates: 30g

- Fat: 10g

- Fiber: 3g

- Sodium: 200mg

Smooth and Refreshing Fruit Smoothie

Preparation Time: 5 minutes

Servings: 1

Ingredients:

- 1 cup mixed berries (strawberries, blueberries, raspberries)

- 1/2 banana

- 1/2 cup plain Greek yogurt

- 1/2 cup orange juice

- 1 tablespoon honey or maple syrup

- Ice cubes (optional)

Directions:

1. Combine all ingredients in a blender.

2. Blend until smooth and creamy.

3. If desired, add ice cubes and blend again until desired consistency is reached.

4. Pour into a glass and enjoy immediately.

Nutrition (per serving):

- Calories: 200

- Protein: 10g

- Carbohydrates: 40g

- Fat: 1g

- Fiber: 5g

- Sodium: 50mg

Creamy Avocado and Banana Smoothie

Preparation Time: 5 minutes

Servings: 1

Ingredients:

- 1/2 ripe avocado

- 1/2 banana

- 1 cup spinach leaves

- 1/2 cup almond milk

- 1 tablespoon honey or maple syrup

- Ice cubes (optional)

Directions:

1. Combine all ingredients in a blender.

2. Blend until smooth and creamy.

3. If desired, add ice cubes and blend again until desired consistency is reached.

4. Pour into a glass and enjoy immediately.

Nutrition (per serving):

- Calories: 250

- Protein: 5g

- Carbohydrates: 30g

- Fat: 15g

- Fiber: 7g

- Sodium: 100mg

Nutritious Green Detox Juice

Preparation Time: 5 minutes

Servings: 1

Ingredients:

- 1 cucumber, peeled and chopped

- 2 celery stalks, chopped

- 1 green apple, cored and chopped

- 1 cup spinach leaves

- 1 tablespoon fresh lemon juice

- 1 cup water or coconut water

- Ice cubes (optional)

Directions:

1. Combine all ingredients in a blender.

2. Blend until smooth.

3. If desired, strain the mixture through a fine-mesh sieve to remove pulp.

4. Pour into a glass and serve immediately over ice cubes, if desired.

 Nutrition (per serving):

- Calories: 100

- Protein: 2g

- Carbohydrates: 25g

- Fat: 1g

- Fiber: 5g

- Sodium: 50mg

Creamy and Energizing Coffee Smoothie

Preparation Time: 5 minutes

Servings: 1

Ingredients:

- 1/2 cup brewed coffee, cooled

- 1/2 cup unsweetened almond milk

- 1/2 banana

- 1 tablespoon almond butter or peanut butter

- 1 tablespoon honey or maple syrup

- Ice cubes (optional)

Directions:

1. Combine all ingredients in a blender.

2. Blend until smooth and creamy.

3. If desired, add ice cubes and blend again until desired consistency is reached.

4. Pour into a glass and enjoy immediately.

Nutrition (per serving):

- Calories: 200

- Protein: 5g

- Carbohydrates: 30g

- Fat: 10g

- Fiber: 3g

- Sodium: 50mg

Refreshing Watermelon and Mint Cooler

Preparation Time: 10 minutes

Servings: 2

Ingredients:

- 4 cups diced seedless watermelon

- 1/4 cup fresh mint leaves

- 1 tablespoon fresh lime juice

- 1 tablespoon honey or agave syrup

- Ice cubes

- Mint sprigs for garnish (optional)

Directions:

1. In a blender, combine diced watermelon, mint leaves, lime juice, and honey.

2. Blend until smooth.

3. Strain the mixture through a fine-mesh sieve to remove any pulp.

4. Pour the strained juice into glasses filled with ice cubes.

5. Garnish with mint sprigs if desired and serve immediately.

Nutrition (per serving):

- Calories: 60

- Protein: 1g

- Carbohydrates: 15g

- Fat: 0g

- Fiber: 1g

- Sodium: 0mg

Nutritious and Creamy Chia Seed Pudding

Preparation Time: 5 minutes (plus overnight soaking)

Servings: 2

Ingredients:

- 1/4 cup chia seeds

- 1 cup unsweetened almond milk

- 1 tablespoon honey or maple syrup

- 1/2 teaspoon vanilla extract

- Fresh fruit for topping (e.g., berries, sliced banana)

- Nuts or seeds for topping (e.g., almonds, pumpkin seeds)

Directions:

1. In a bowl, whisk together chia seeds, almond milk, honey, and vanilla extract.

2. Cover and refrigerate overnight, or for at least 4 hours, until the mixture thickens and forms a pudding-like consistency.

3. Stir well before serving and add more almond milk if desired to adjust consistency.

4. Divide the pudding into serving dishes and top with fresh fruit, nuts, or seeds.

Nutrition (per serving):

- Calories: 150

- Protein: 4g

- Carbohydrates: 20g

- Fat: 6g

- Fiber: 8g

- Sodium: 80mg

Smooth and Creamy Yogurt Shake

Preparation Time: 5 minutes

Servings:1

Ingredients:

- 1 cup Greek yogurt

- 1/2 cup milk of choice (e.g., almond milk, soy milk)

- 1/2 banana

- 1 tablespoon honey or maple syrup

- 1/2 teaspoon vanilla extract

- Ice cubes (optional)

Directions:

1. Combine all ingredients in a blender.

2. Blend until smooth and creamy.

3. If desired, add ice cubes and blend again until desired consistency is reached.

4. Pour into a glass and enjoy immediately.

Nutrition (per serving):

- Calories: 300

- Protein: 25g

- Carbohydrates: 40g

- Fat: 5g

- Fiber: 2g

- Sodium: 150mg

Preparation Time: 5 minutes

Servings: 1

Ingredients:

- 1 cup spinach leaves

- 1/2 ripe avocado

- 1/2 banana

- 1/2 cup pineapple chunks

- 1 tablespoon chia seeds

- 1 cup coconut water

- Ice cubes (optional)

Directions:

1. Combine all ingredients in a blender.

2. Blend until smooth.

3. If desired, add ice cubes and blend again until desired consistency is reached.

4. Pour into a glass and enjoy immediately.

Nutrition (per serving):

- Calories: 250

- Protein: 5g

- Carbohydrates: 30g

- Fat: 15g

- Fiber: 10g

- Sodium: 150mg

Creamy and Refreshing Mango Lassi

Preparation Time: 5 minutes

Servings: 2

Ingredients:

- 1 cup ripe mango chunks

- 1 cup plain Greek yogurt

- 1/2 cup milk of choice (e.g., almond milk, coconut milk)

- 1 tablespoon honey or maple syrup

- 1/4 teaspoon ground cardamom (optional)

- Ice cubes (optional)

- Sliced mango for garnish (optional)

Directions:

1. In a blender, combine mango chunks, Greek yogurt, milk, honey, and ground cardamom.

2. Blend until smooth and creamy.

3. If desired, add ice cubes and blend again until desired consistency is reached.

4. Pour into glasses, garnish with sliced mango if desired, and serve immediately.

Nutrition (per serving):

- Calories: 200

- Protein: 10g

- Carbohydrates: 30g

- Fat: 5g

- Fiber: 2g

- Sodium: 80mg

Nutritious and Creamy Oatmeal Smoothie

Preparation Time: 5 minutes

Servings: 1

Ingredients:

- 1/2 cup rolled oats

- 1/2 banana

- 1 tablespoon peanut butter or almond butter

- 1 tablespoon honey or maple syrup

- 1/2 cup plain Greek yogurt

- 1/2 cup milk of choice (e.g., almond milk, oat milk)

- Ice cubes (optional)

- Pinch of cinnamon (optional)

Directions:

1. In a blender, combine rolled oats, banana, peanut butter, honey, Greek yogurt, and milk.

2. Blend until smooth and creamy.

3. If desired, add ice cubes and blend again until desired consistency is reached.

4. Pour into a glass, sprinkle with a pinch of cinnamon if desired, and serve immediately.

Nutrition (per serving):

- Calories: 350

- Protein: 15g

- Carbohydrates: 50g

- Fat: 10g

- Fiber: 5g

- Sodium: 100mg

Refreshing Cucumber and Lemon Infused Water

Preparation Time: 5 minutes (plus chilling time)

Servings: 2

Ingredients:

- 4 cups water

- 1 cucumber, thinly sliced

- 1 lemon, thinly sliced

- Fresh mint leaves

- Ice cubes (optional)

Directions:

1. In a pitcher, combine water, cucumber slices, lemon slices, and fresh mint leaves.

2. Chill in the refrigerator for at least 1 hour to allow the flavors to infuse.

3. Serve over ice cubes if desired.

Nutrition (per serving):

- Calories: 0

- Protein: 0g

- Carbohydrates: 0g

- Fat: 0g

- Fiber: 0g

- Sodium: 0mg

Preparation Time: 5 minutes

Servings: 1

Ingredients:

- 1 cup unsweetened almond milk

- 1/2 banana

- 1 tablespoon almond butter

- 1 tablespoon honey or maple syrup

- 1/2 teaspoon vanilla extract

- Ice cubes (optional)

Directions:

1. In a blender, combine almond milk, banana, almond butter, honey, and vanilla extract.

2. Blend until smooth and creamy.

3. If desired, add ice cubes and blend again until desired consistency is reached.

4. Pour into a glass and serve immediately.

Nutrition (per serving):

- Calories: 250

- Protein: 5g

- Carbohydrates: 30g

- Fat: 12g

- Fiber: 3g

- Sodium: 150mg

Preparation Time: 5 minutes

Servings: 1

Ingredients:

- 1/2 cup mixed berries (strawberries, blueberries, raspberries)

- 1/2 banana

- 1/2 cup plain Greek yogurt

- 1/2 cup milk of choice (e.g., almond milk, soy milk)

- 1 tablespoon honey or maple syrup

- Ice cubes (optional)

Directions:

1. In a blender, combine mixed berries, banana, Greek yogurt, milk, and honey.

2. Blend until smooth and creamy.

3. If desired, add ice cubes and blend again until desired consistency is reached.

4. Pour into a glass and serve immediately.

Nutrition (per serving):

- Calories: 200

- Protein: 10g

- Carbohydrates: 35g

- Fat: 2g

- Fiber: 5g

- Sodium: 50mg

Nutritious and Creamy Peanut Butter Banana Shake

Preparation Time: 5 minutes

Servings: 1

Ingredients:

- 1/2 banana

- 1 tablespoon peanut butter

- 1 cup milk of choice (e.g., almond milk, cow's milk)

- 1 tablespoon honey or maple syrup

- Ice cubes (optional)

Directions:

1. In a blender, combine banana, peanut butter, milk, and honey.

2. Blend until smooth and creamy.

3. If desired, add ice cubes and blend again until desired consistency is reached.

4. Pour into a glass and serve immediately.

Nutrition (per serving):

- Calories: 300

- Protein: 10g

- Carbohydrates: 40g

- Fat: 12g

- Fiber: 3g

- Sodium: 150mg

Refreshing and Hydrating Coconut Water

Preparation Time: 5 minutes

Servings: 1

Ingredients:

- 1 cup coconut water

- Ice cubes (optional)

- Lemon or lime slices for garnish (optional)

- Mint leaves for garnish (optional)

Directions:

1. Pour coconut water into a glass.

2. Add ice cubes if desired.

3. Garnish with lemon or lime slices and mint leaves if desired.

4. Serve immediately and enjoy the refreshing drink.

Nutrition (per serving):

- Calories: 45

- Protein: 0g

- Carbohydrates: 11g

- Fat: 0g

- Fiber: 0g

- Sodium: 60mg

Preparation Time: 5 minutes

Servings: 1

Ingredients:

- 1/2 cup Greek yogurt

- 1/2 cup frozen mixed berries (strawberries, blueberries, raspberries)

- 1/2 banana

- 1 tablespoon honey or maple syrup

- 1/2 cup milk of choice (e.g., almond milk, cow's milk)

- Ice cubes (optional)

Directions:

1. In a blender, combine Greek yogurt, frozen mixed berries, banana, honey, and milk.

2. Blend until smooth and creamy.

3. If desired, add ice cubes and blend again until desired consistency is reached.

4. Pour into a glass and serve immediately.

Nutrition (per serving):

- Calories: 250

- Protein: 15g

- Carbohydrates: 40g

- Fat: 4g

- Fiber: 5g

- Sodium: 90mg

Energizing and Nutritious Matcha Green Tea Latte

Preparation Time:5 minutes

Servings: 1

Ingredients:

- 1 teaspoon matcha green tea powder

- 1 cup milk of choice (e.g., almond milk, cow's milk)

- 1 tablespoon honey or maple syrup

- Ice cubes (optional)

Directions:

1. In a small bowl, whisk matcha green tea powder with a little bit of hot water until smooth.

2. In a glass, combine the matcha mixture, milk, and honey.

3. Stir well until combined.

4. If desired, add ice cubes to chill the latte.

5. Serve immediately and enjoy the energizing drink.

Nutrition (per serving):

- Calories: 100

- Protein: 7g

- Carbohydrates: 20g

- Fat: 1g

- Fiber: 1g

- Sodium: 120mg

Preparation Time: 5 minutes

Servings: 1

Ingredients:

- 1 cup water

- 1/2 lemon, thinly sliced

- 1-inch piece of ginger, thinly sliced

- Fresh mint leaves (optional)

- Ice cubes (optional)

Directions:

1. In a glass, combine water, lemon slices, and ginger slices.

2. Add fresh mint leaves if desired.

3. If desired, add ice cubes to chill the water.

4. Stir well and let it sit for a few minutes to allow the flavors to infuse.

5. Serve immediately and enjoy the refreshing and detoxifying drink.

Nutrition (per serving):

- Calories: 0

- Protein: 0g

- Carbohydrates: 0g

- Fat: 0g

- Fiber: 0g

- Sodium: 0mg

Chapter 7:

CONCLUSION

Celebrating Your Journey with Dysphagia

Living with dysphagia, a condition that affects swallowing, can present unique challenges. However, it's important to recognize and celebrate your journey as you navigate through these difficulties. In this chapter, we'll explore ways to embrace your experiences and find joy along the way.

1. Acknowledge Your Strengths:

Take a moment to recognize the strength and resilience you've demonstrated in managing dysphagia. Celebrate your ability to adapt and find new ways to enjoy food and beverages. Embrace the progress you've made and the lessons you've learned.

2. Discover New Culinary Experiences:

While dysphagia may require dietary modifications, it doesn't mean you can't enjoy delicious meals. Explore recipes and techniques that cater to your needs, such as pureed or soft foods. Engage in the creative process of preparing meals and savor the flavors and textures that bring you joy.

3. Share Your Story:

Consider sharing your dysphagia journey with others. Whether it's through conversations with friends and family or participating in support groups, sharing your experiences can increase awareness and understanding. It may also inspire and encourage others who are going through similar challenges.

4. Set Achievable Goals:

Celebrate milestones along your journey by setting achievable goals related to your dysphagia management. It could be as simple as trying a new food or successfully completing a swallowing exercise. Recognize the progress you've made and celebrate each step forward.

5. Practice Self-Care:

Taking care of yourself is crucial throughout your dysphagia journey. Celebrate by engaging in activities that promote your well-being, such as practicing relaxation techniques, pursuing hobbies, or indulging in self-care rituals. Remember to prioritize your physical, emotional, and mental health.

Final Thoughts and Encouragement

As you reach the end of this guide, it's important to reflect on your journey with dysphagia and find encouragement to continue moving forward. Remember, you are not alone in facing these challenges, and there is support available to help you thrive. This final chapter offers some closing thoughts and words of encouragement.

1. Stay Positive and Resilient:

Maintain a positive mindset and focus on your strengths and achievements. Recognize that managing dysphagia requires resilience and adaptability, and celebrate the progress you've made. Embrace the challenges as opportunities for growth and continue to navigate your journey with determination.

2. Seek Support and Connection:

Remember to lean on your support network. Reach out to friends, family, and support groups to share your experiences, seek guidance, and find emotional support. Connecting with others who understand your journey can provide a sense of belonging and encouragement.

3. Advocate for Yourself:

Be an advocate for your own needs and well-being. Communicate openly with your healthcare team, voice your concerns, and actively participate in your treatment plan. Your input and insights are valuable in shaping your dysphagia management journey.

4. Celebrate Every Milestone:

Take the time to celebrate every milestone, no matter how small it may seem. Each achievement, whether it's trying a new food or mastering a swallowing exercise, is a step forward in your journey. Celebrate your progress and use it as motivation to keep pushing forward.

5. Embrace the Joy of Eating:

While dysphagia may bring challenges to mealtimes, remember to find joy in the act of eating. Explore new flavors, savor each bite, and appreciate the nourishment and pleasure that food brings. Focus on the sensory experience and the connections it fosters with others.

In conclusion, your journey with dysphagia is unique, and it requires patience, perseverance, and a willingness to explore new possibilities. Embrace the resources available to you, stay connected with others, and celebrate your progress along the way. With time, adaptability, and support, you can continue to find satisfaction and joy in your relationship with food.

9 798327 998438